ALSO BY DONNA HUSTON MURRAY

The Ginger Barnes Main Line Mysteries:

THE MAIN LINE IS MURDER

FINAL ARRANGEMENTS

SCHOOL OF HARD KNOCKS

NO BONES ABOUT IT

A SCORE TO SETTLE

FAREWELL PERFORMANCE

LIE LIKE A RUG

Please feel free to contact the author
@**www.donnahustonmurray.com**

ISBN: 978-0-9856880-4-2

Dedicated to my wonderful mentors:
Harriet Mae Savitz and Barbara Bates

Chapter 1

Holding myself together is tough, but if Corinne's daughter can do it, I damn well better. Distraction. That's what I need, a distraction.

All sorts of people are here to pay their respects, but middle-aged mourners and upward predominate–partly because Corinne's own age was fifty-seven, but also because of her profession. I'm guessing she counseled most of the congregation through their own cancer ordeal.

I'm only thirty, but we met that way, too. I've also lived under her roof a little over four years, but probably not much longer. It's Nina's roof now.

As if she heard her name, Corinne's daughter twists around in her front-row seat. For a moment she basks in the sympathy wafting her way; but then she sees me, and her head snaps forward so fast that wiry hair of hers actually bounces.

The florid-faced clergyman steps up to the pulpit. "We have gathered here today to honor a woman who…"

I tune out his soporific voice, stare at the stained-glass window, make note of a loose comb in a woman's frizzy hairdo, and before I know it greetings are being exchanged, backs patted, coats gathered, purses, programs with Corinne's picture and prayers typed in italics.

We adjourn to the annex community room where tables covered with yellow paper line up in rows, food and drink on three perpendicular to the rest.

Nina is surrounded, but I catch her daughter Jilly's eye. A soft-bodied eight-year-old with self-esteem issues, this is surely her first funeral. She sends me a brave smile, and I nod my encouragement. She may be Nina's only child, but she has a life away from her mother, too. She'll be alright.

I've sidled up to my honorary uncles Norman and Tom, two of my dad's dearest friends.

"Nice homily," Norman remarks.

Tom just sipped some fruit punch, so he grunts his agreement. Then he asks, "What did you think, Beanie?" My father's endearment: Lauren Louise Beck, LLBean...

I open my mouth, but that's as far as I get. Nina is storming toward me, fists clenched, face aflame. A chair falls by the wayside. "You," she shouts, "you've got a nerve."

The room goes silent. Faces gape and stare.

"You miserable, goddamn *bitch*. You killed my *mother*. I can't believe you're here, you you you *MURDERER!*" Hands covering her face, Nina crumbles into the arms of a man in a business suit, the despised ex-husband.

"Now, Nina," he murmurs. "You don't really mean..."

Her head snaps up. "Oh yes I do," she shouts even louder. Then she wrestles out of his grasp, clenches her fists, growls through her teeth.

The uncles and I have backed up so far we're literally against the cement-block wall. The whole room is holding its breath.

"Nina, really." I pat the air. "You're upset. You don't know what you're saying."

"The hell I don't." The whites of her eyes are so exposed she looks rabid. "You're going to jail for a long, long time, Lauren Beck..."

Many of the onlookers are friends of my family. Others know the Beck name from dad's farm or his real estate dealings, or they remember my brother from the sports page back when he made All-American in lacrosse.

Maybe I arrested somebody's husband or son for something or other, or ticketed them for speeding when I was back on the job.

Nobody here will forget me now. Never mind that I'm innocent; I've just become the OJ Simpson of Landis, Pennsylvania.

Pointing toward the door, Nina's vicious "GET OUT!" lands on me like spit.

Norman steps forward, but I halt him with my arm. "She's just upset," I tell the old bulldog. "I'll be okay."

But I won't. My dad's friend knows it, and I know it; but he backs off anyhow. What other choice does he have?

The annex door clunks shut behind me. Nina's shocker has temporarily put my grief at bay, but I can't remember where I left my Miata. Doesn't matter though; there's an unmarked car at the curb.

Wearing softened designer jeans, a tweed sport coat, and no particular expression, Scarp Poletta summons me with a lift of his chin. As I plod down the cement steps, he opens the passenger door more like a gentleman than a homicide cop.

When we're eye to eye, I finally ask. "Is this our first date, or are you here to arrest me?"

Chapter 2

Amazing. Until last week I hadn't crossed paths with Scarp Poletta for years, and surprise, surprise, here he is again...during working hours for a homicide detective...and I've just been accused of murder.

"You didn't answer my question," I remind him.

"Just a friendly ride...for now," he answers. Not a huge relief, but better than a poke in the eye.

Slipping past him into the passenger seat, I catch a whiff of ocean spray with a hint of cinnamon bagel, and I can't help thinking about our previous encounter.

IT HAD been an exceptionally bad day for Corinne. Because she hadn't needed nausea medicine for her chemo before, she received it late. Too late. When I got home from work, Nina was up to her ears in alligators. She actually allowed me to help put her mother to bed, clean the powder room, and throw some soiled laundry in the washer. I also packed Jilly for a stay with her father, took her to McDonald's for dinner, and dropped her off. When I got back, Nina was draped across the chintz sofa staring at a glass of merlot.

I helped myself to a nearby chair. "Listen," I said. "I know how rough this is. I've been there, remember? So how about we smoke the peace pipe here and now and do this together?"

"Fuck off," she shot back. Then she curled up to cry.

Not much I could say to that.

I trudged up the two flights to my attic loft, struggled through a shower, put on jeans and a turtleneck, then grabbed my coat. For the first time in four years I was going to a bar.

Another woman would have invited a girlfriend to join her, but I'd been out of circulation so long I had nobody to call. So it would be Casey's Tavern, the cop bar in Landis I'd frequented back on the job. There at least I stood a chance of meeting up with one or two of my former co-workers.

I steered into a slot thirty-yards from the entrance then trotted through the evening chill across smooth new macadam. Except for the neon Coors and Budweiser signs, Casey's low, brick building might have housed auto parts. A framed menu by the door told me my old haunt served food now; and inside—inside were more women than ever before, fifteen at least mingling with the forty or so men. Probably spoke well for the food.

I'd almost forgotten happy-hour noise—the boisterous conversations, dishes being bussed, bottles clinking, cheers or groans depending on what the Flyers had just done on the huge HD TV. The oblong bar to the left and the thick pine tabletops were the same. So was the welcoming fragrance of spilled beer. I didn't recognize any of the bartenders.

Hands in my hip pockets, neck craning as if I were looking for someone, I took a couple of tentative steps inside. I had on my last clean turtleneck, which happened to be red, and an overweight boozer swiveled on his barstool to check me out. Then a waitress looked through me as she wove by with six long neck bottles on a tray. Laughter erupted across the room, then cheers for a Flyers save.

No pairs of women at the bar for me to stand near, no singles of any sort. In less than a minute my palms were wet and my smile felt like a plaster cast. I decided I was either crazy or desperate to be there. Maybe both.

Then a hearty baritone called out, "Lauren Beck, you bitch, you never call, you never write. Get the hell over here and give me a kiss."

"Garry, you old dog," I responded. "Arlene kick you out again?"

"Very funny." He patted the seat of the empty chair beside him.

"That's my exit line," his drinking companion announced, throwing some bills down next to a dirty plate. "See you in the morning, Gar. Nice to meet ya, hon, whoever you are."

"Oh, hell." Garry threw out a name I didn't catch in the noise, Ron something. We shook, then he shambled off toward the door.

"Beer?" my old friend offered. His hairline had receded a bit, and he was carrying more weight around the middle. I thought he looked mellower, a little more content with the world.

"Yes, please," I said regarding the beer. "So how is Arlene?"

The cop's eyes sparkled, and his lips eased into a slow smile. "She's splendid, thank you very much."

"So what the hell are you doing here?"

Garry leaned onto the broad round table and began to pick at the label on his Miller Lite. "Cosmetics party, can you believe it?"

I gave that more laugh than it deserved while the hockey crowd groaned.

Garry waited out the noise with a steady gaze. Then he said, "You look good, Lauren. How you doin'?"

I was so touched that I told him the truth. "Cured, Gar. Can you believe it?"

I'd been cancer-free more than four years; and about then Hodgkins survivors can pretty much relax about a recurrence. Yet this was the first time I'd said as much out loud, and it felt a little as if I were tempting fate.

"Seriously?"

"Yeah. Isn't it great?" It was. And there went the last of my doubts. *Face it, Lauren, you're a very lucky girl.*

Garry saw what I was thinking and grinned. "You comin' back?"

"Doubtful. I just started with AIA this week. SIU" The Amalgamated Insurance Association of North America's Special Investigative Unit.

"Good for you, girl. Go get 'em." What an adorable man.

We spent the better part of a beer catching up on things—Arlene and the kids, what Garry was doing (he'd switched to trapping pedophiles via the internet). I touched on my old part-time job doing background checks for Allstate's Directors and Officers' policies from home.

"Something to keep body and soul together," Garry observed with an approving nod.

"Exactly. Now I'm trying to help out with my landlady's chemo treatments, but her daughter's giving me a hard time."

"Sounds like she's more than just a landlady."

"You always did catch on quick."

I explained about Corinne starting out as my cancer counselor and almost becoming much more. "She took me in to nurse me through the Hodgkins when she and Dad were an item. They didn't last, but Corinne and I did." I shrugged. "We get along, and I think she's glad for the rent. I try to help out however I can." When Nina let me

I was about to start in on the weather; but that's when Scarp Poletta showed up, the third empty plate at the table

He explained his absence with a mumbled, "Lawyer bought me a drink." Then he gave me a long look and a throaty, "Hello."

"Hi," I replied.

I won't say Poletta is tall, dark and handsome, because these days five-ten is considered average height. Dark, yes, and built thick and solid as a plow-horse, but nobody would call him pretty. Too many creases in his face, for one thing.

"You two know each other?" Garry inquired.

I said, "Sort of."

Poletta said, "Not well." Then he focused those chocolate brown eyes right on me. "Heard you were sick," he stated carefully. "Good to see you out and about."

"Thanks." I felt hot to the roots of my hair and desperately hoped it didn't show.

"Please sit," Scarp remarked, which was when I realized I was standing.

The homicide detective watched me settle down with twitching lips. Lord only knows what he was thinking, but me? I was concentrating on how his nose angled sharply to the left, his dark, herringbone eyebrows, and his narrow forehead. Attractive as hell, but, thank God, not beautiful. Brent W. Cahill's face had been picture perfect, so now I preferred almost anything else.

"You still with Rainy McQuinn?" I inquired, Rainy McQuinn being a notorious basket case. Scarp and she had been on again/off again forever.

When he stopped laughing, I said, "Well, are you?" Some things you just plain need to know.

"Yeah," he admitted. "Although sometimes I wonder why. What about you?"

"What about me?"

He lifted my left hand. "You give up on that reporter? Whatisname?"

"Brent Cahill. And the answer is no. He gave up on me when I was diagnosed with cancer."

Scarp looked truly shocked. For a minute he couldn't even speak.

"It's okay. I'm over it. All of it. I'm over everything." I'd be damned if I was going to admit that I wasn't back up to speed in the dating department.

Garry nodded his approval, and the waitress brought another round. I waved mine away, though, being as how I was quite the health nut now. I was also thinking how embarrassing it would be to get pulled over by one of my former co-workers, even if a bunch of them were presently drinking plenty more than me.

Scarp cocked one of those bushy eyebrows. "Then you won't mind if I tell you he's right over there."

I exhaled as if I'd been sucker punched and ducked my head. Then I squinted through the crowd to see if Scarp was messing with me.

Unfortunately, the man did not lie. There big as life and twice as beautiful was Brent W. Cahill, TV news anchor and ex-love of my life, holding a beer by the throat and enthralling another man and a woman with some scintillating story. The three of them reared back with laughter, but no one laughed more heartily than Brent. Even dressed in oxford cloth and tweed his baseball-pitcher build and blond good looks blended with the Casey's crowd much better than I ever had.

"Shit," Garry muttered. Scarp was already grinning at my expense. "What's that asshole doing here?"

The answer was so simple that I waved it off.

Brent adored Casey's. We used to stop in once or twice a week, usually at his suggestion. Naively, I imagined that mingling with my fellow cops was a way for him to learn more about my work and, by extension, about me. Later—

some would say too late—I realized he was cultivating sources. He was a reporter, after all.

I glanced at Garry, dear married Garry, the honorable knight who had rescued my evening, then at Scarp, as tempting as the steak on your neighbor's grill, and decided I wasn't having fun anymore.

"G'night, guys," I told them as I reached for my wallet.

Later I would remember that as the night I found our mail slit open. Nina had been tending her mother all day and wouldn't have checked the box, so I slipped through the quiet house toward the front door, past kitchen shelves loaded with bobble-heads and cookie-jars, between the living room sofa and coffee table and around the silent TV. My beer with the guys had made me nostalgic and sentimental, so I allowed myself to hope for something from my father–a news clipping, a recipe, a joke.

Flipping on the porch light, I dug out the handful of grocery-store fliers and junk. My credit card and phone bills were there, too, and a some medical correspondence addressed to Corinne. I figured the elderly woman next door had accidentally opened some misdirected mail; but when the other stuff started happening, I finally asked.

It hadn't been her.

Chapter 3

Outside the church Scarp tells me, "Buckle up," with an amused smirk that douses my libido.

Fastening my seat belt takes three tries because my hands are so slippery, and I don't even ask where we're going for the first mile because I'm afraid I might hurl.

"Where would you like to go?" he inquires.

Anywhere but jail.

"Montana" I tell him, "or maybe Wyoming. Someplace with a small population. My luck with people hasn't been so hot lately."

He nods as if he isn't surprised, so I mention my second choice. "I could use a cup of coffee."

"That I can do." He does a U turn back toward the Glendenning countryside.

I'm not aware of any coffee shops out there, but the police lockup is steadily growing further away, so I zip my lip.

"So," he says with a sideways glance. "What happened back there?"

I shrug and try a que-cera-cera smile. "High noon, except I forgot my gun."

Scarp's right eyebrow lifts. Then he passes a slowpoke and settles back in lane before he gives me the news flash. "You realize I'm here in an official capacity. So maybe you better ease off on the humor."

"Would that be 'read me my rights' official capacity, or 'protect me from that madwoman' official capacity?"

His turn to shrug. "Just tell me straight. What happened?"

"Nina freaked out and accused me of killing her mother. It was a helluva scene. Everybody heard her." I can still feel the stares scorching my skin.

We are now square in the middle of my childhood world–lush Pennsylvania farmland with cows huffing into the humid November air. Scarp, as in "You naughty little scarper," eases the car into a grassy gutter and steps on the parking brake. He reaches behind him for an old-fashioned glass-lined thermos, fills the red lid with black coffee, and hands it to me.

"Starbucks," he brags, and I raise the cup in a toast. I'm usually a cream and sugar customer, but the warmth couldn't be any more welcome and the flavor is quite acceptable. I offer my captor a sip.

He ignores me, rests his arm on the back of the seat before twisting my way.

"On Monday Nina got an anonymous phone call telling her you murdered her mother. She phoned the Landis police. They called the District Attorney, and he handed the case to me."

"Case? There is no case."

Scarp shoots me a look, and then I remember. Unless a crime is immediately obvious, most investigations begin with a thread equally as thin.

I force myself to breathe. "What did the tip say?"

"You know I can't tell you that."

"How about this? I wasn't anywhere near the hospital when Corinne died."

Scarp does another, smaller shrug. "I know. I talked to Dr. Brooks this morning. He said he called the number you gave him soon after Mrs. Wilder passed away. You didn't return his call."

I'm churning inside, dying to defend myself anyway I can, but there's a warning flag flapping in my face. During

Corinne's final horrible quest for air I, too, longed for a handy bystander to blame. As a result, I insulted a woman who'd simply been doing her job—dispensing the hospital's supply of drugs.

Yet even if it was grief speaking, Scarp will approach Nina's accusation like the professional investigator he is, so I need to gather my wits and do the same. Once the impression of guilt settles in, it's damn near impossible to outlive the stigma.

Which prompts another possibility. It could be argued that the stress of the funeral caused Nina's self-control to snap exactly when it damaged me most—but I wasn't buying. Yes, we avoided each other all week; but the handful of times we did cross paths I sensed nothing close to the venom she slung my way half an hour ago. So either she's a master at deception, or she hates me even more than I suspected. Maybe both.

And now I'm a bona fide murder suspect. Scarp knows I wasn't anywhere near Corinne when she died, so the premise must be that I introduced some slow-acting poison or drug into her IV drip to allow time for an alibi. Unfortunately, proving or disproving that theory would require an autopsy, and Corinne's remains have already been cremated.

I shake my head and take a deep breath. "I'm screwed, aren't I?"

Scarp interrupts his own reflections to face me again. "Not necessarily." His demeanor shows me he isn't kidding around and neither is the District Attorney.

And yet we're out here in the middle of Glendenning county—my turf—rather than in an interrogation room at the county lockup. Until some sort of tangible evidence turns up, it appears that I'm being given the benefit of a doubt.

"Why not necessarily?" I ask. "What've you got?"

Scarp lifts one of his beautiful shoulders, a shoulder that, another time another place, I would love to bite. "The nurse and the doctor signed off on pneumonia."

Finally, a straw to grasp. "So you don't really have anything?"

The homicide detective shifts around again, giving me a hormone surge. "Not really," he agrees. "But neither do you."

Too true. I have no ammunition except the fact that I adored Corinne, and that could be argued away with one word—*euthanasia*. Considering our history, it would be easy to persuade a jury that I couldn't stand to see her suffer, that my empathy was so great I felt compelled to end her life. I could swear I was innocent until the cows came home, but who would listen?

While I sip at the coffee, Scarp and I throw around a few ideas, none of them much help; and finally the caffeine and the conversation begin to clear my head. I ask whether anyone is looking into Nina's phone records to check if she got a call at the time she said she did.

"She claims she got the tip Monday morning at her mother's house, but condolence calls came in all day. No way of knowing what was said during any of those conversations."

Personally, I'm torn between believing there was a phony tip and believing that Nina wrote her own script. With her, either seemed possible.

I open my car door and toss the coffee dregs into the grass.

"You need lunch?" my old acquaintance inquires as he reaches for the ignition key.

"God, no," I reply. "My stomach wouldn't know what to do with food right now."

"Tomorrow?"

While I wonder whether or not to be pleased by the invitation, Scarp turns the car around and settles into a slow cruise toward town.

"Are you really interested?" I ask at last, "or are you afraid to let me out of your sight?"

Poletta opts for inscrutable silence, so I tell him no thanks, that I'd rather not be accused of murder just to spice up my social life.

More silence, punctuated by an irritating smirk. Maybe Rainy can have this one, after all. So what if he has eyes like a golden retriever and thighs like granite? I've taken the cure. Not interested. No thank you.

"Where to then?" he inquires mildly.

"Pick up my car, I guess." The funeral luncheon will be winding down, but I may be able to grab my running shoes and get out of the house before Nina returns home.

Home. Without Corinne it no longer feels like home. Yet all my stuff is there, and my rent is paid up for a couple more weeks. Soon I'll have to do something about finding a new place, but short term I figure I'll just tread lightly. Eat out. Keep my comings and goings to a minimum. Like that.

Right now, however, I want to check on my Glock. When I learned that Nina and Jilly were moving in, I hid it on the rafter above my bed. Now I want to get it out of the house altogether. Maybe carry it in my car.

Or, better yet, at the small of my back.

Chapter 4

The pavement hammers the tenseness from my body one stride at a time while split-level houses and modest colonials blur past my eyes. So familiar is my route that only things in motion register–the car turning left on Hobbs, the new mother pushing a stroller. The sidewalk jostles her red-cheeked boy so violently he can scarcely stay in his seat, but the mother is oblivious. She smiles me a hello nod that seems to say, "I'm going to ruin this kid with my good intentions, just try and stop me."

At least his therapist will know where to start. For Nina I can only guess at divorce–her mother's when she was little, then her own five years ago. I only recently became her scapegoat, but for her mother's sake I'm prepared to endure whatever I must from the woman.

The sun offers only a half-hearted warmth; but as I begin to clock the miles, I welcome the chill. Four or five is my habit; but endorphins have summoned up my first success at work, and the farther I run the more I view my small victory in a new and disturbing light. Lost in the mental debate I press on past the water tower all the way to the Little League field.

If Nina actually received that incriminating phone call, it meant somebody else harbored a healthy animosity toward me. My ex-fiance had already done his worst, and until recently I'd been living like a recluse, so the candidate pool was pretty shallow. The only new contacts were at my job, which, I admit, deprived people of money they honestly, or *dishonestly*, felt they deserved. A few inquiries online or around town and my life was an open book. Even a casual water-cooler conversation with my boss could have elicited enough about me to put my neck in Nina's noose. Yet no particular incident stood out, so I started my mental recap with Tuesday, my second day at AIA.

I HAD been passing by my supervisor's ninth-floor, glass-enclosed office with a fresh mug of coffee when David Willard, never Dave, *oh-heavens-no,* reeled me in with a hand wave.

Crowding the threshold was a lumbering lout of a man with black fishhook sideburns, protruding lips, and a large fleshy nose. Oblivious to my approach, he said, "About the Young/Burton claim. Can we...?"

"Hold that thought, Bob," David interrupted. "I'd like you to meet Lauren Beck, our new hire. Lauren, this is Bob Battersby, probably our biggest producer." The boss's shoulders pulled back with pride, and his cheeks bloomed pink enough to clash with his limp blond hair. Not the athletic sort, our David. A target for bullies, perhaps, in his not-too-distant youth.

Battersby's raw-oyster eyes washed over me. "Yeh, hello," he said, "Nice to meetcha." Then he attempted to dismiss me with a brief, skin-deep smile.

I knew his type from back on the job–an old-school cop who would give a female investigator her props about when AIA starts to pay overtime. Run amok, Battersby's outdated attitude could ruin an otherwise placid work environment.

"Have a seat, Bob," David suggested. "You, too, Lauren. Maybe you can help."

Battersby took the closest visitor's chair for himself and cringed when I squeezed past to get to the other.

"A closed head injury," David began to fill me in. "Fellow claiming permanent mental deficiency as a result of being hit on the head by a golf club."

"Guess that would do it," I remarked, and Bob-darling rolled his eyes.

David tented his fingers on his desk to use for punctuation. "A falling golf club, Lauren." Tap and pause. "The insured took his new putter to his patio table to show a friend," tap, "leaned it against a porch railing while he was eating lunch," tap, "then bumped it with his chair when he stood up." Double tap and a hand spread. "It was an accident, Lauren. The putter fell through the railing and hit another Merlin Heights member on the head."

Bob raked his hair and scowled. "Unfortunately, my outside source didn't turn up a damn thing."

"Outside source?"

Bob shot David a critical glance. "We can't be everyplace at once," he informed me, "so we outsource our surveillances."

"Good to know, Bob." Didn't get to that *on my first day,* Bob. "Is the PI one you trust?"

Battersby's eyes narrowed. "We trust all our sub-contractors."

Our boss tilted his head and waved a hand about ear level. "Not so quick, Bob," he protested. "You said yourself the guy's faking. Now which is it? Do you think he's faking or not?"

"Faking. Definitely faking. But we can't prove it."

"You mean we haven't proven it yet."

"Fine. You want me to shelve everything else and stick to the old bastard like toilet paper? We already paid Klein to do that, and he came up with buptkus."

"No, no," David's voice was mollifying now. "That's why I asked Lauren in here." He turned to me. "How would you handle this?"

I glanced from one man to the other. David looked ridiculously hopeful and eager, as if he expected me to come up with something brilliant; and Bob appeared to be praying I wouldn't. The perfect no-win situation.

I had to say something, so I said, "I guess I'd look over the surveillance report again. Maybe retrace some of the, uh, victim's steps myself, see if the PI missed anything."

It was pretty elementary stuff, but David swelled with paternal pride. "Sounds good to me." He clapped his hands together with a resounding smack then rubbed away the sting. "Sound good to you, Bob?"

"I suppose we don't have anything to lose."

"Just two million!" David replied. "Lauren, can you get right on it?"

I said, "Sure," but I felt right and truly snookered. As a training exercise, this was one hundred percent ass-backward; but as an opportunity to make me look incompetent, it took the prize. I could disappoint my new boss and justify Bob's pin-headed prejudice all at once.

With no other choice, I accepted the folder David handed me.

The company Taurus I inherited from my predecessor smelled like an ashtray, so I cracked a window and let the damp breeze have its way with my streaky blonde curls. Blessing EZ-Pass, I joined the early afternoon throng heading east, took the Pennsylvania turnpike bridge across the Delaware River, then headed north on the Jersey turnpike until I reached the Mount Holly Interchange. From there, my company's aged GPS steered me through a series of local roads toward Cranbury, and, to my amazement, exactly where I needed to go.

The Merlin Heights Country Club is old as a musket and prettier than a southern mansion. Open white board fencing allows non-members to view jade fairways studded with emerald greens while subtly reminding us that we may not walk on the grass. I parked in a visitor's slot and let myself into the gray stone clubhouse through two enormous double doors.

The dining room was in the back, where I found a cute, six-foot-two waiter setting out flatware. I explained who I was and what I needed, and the young man's lips twitched ever so slightly. Amused by an old man going to the emergency room? Unlikely. There was a certain look in his eye, the stirring of an old memory; he was flirting with me. He was too young, of course, but I couldn't help putting a little extra warmth into my words. "You were here that day?"

"Yes ma'm."

Ma'm? Oh. He was teasing me for responding, which made me laugh. "Great," I said. "Then you can show me where Mr. Young was sitting when the accident occurred."

"Certainly. Right this way."

I followed him onto a patio that spanned the width of the building. Down below an old duffer in a yellow windbreaker missed a putt on the eighteenth green.

"Over here, Ms. Beck." The waiter pointed to a chair backing up to a long row of cement balustrades topped with wooden railing.

Having no idea what Bob Battersby had already done, it made sense to start from scratch. That meant photographs and measurements in case the matter went to trial.

"So Mr. Young leaned his putter here," I thought out loud. "Then when he finished lunch, he stood up, knocked the putter through the railing, and it landed," I peered over the edge at an apron of macadam, "down there."

"That's about it," the waiter agreed. His dark eyes glowed with the dangerous intelligence of a guy I dated in college, and for a second all I could think of was locked bedroom doors and boozy breath.

Damn. Maybe I really should put myself out there again.

I extended my metal measuring tape down to the ground, wrote a note, then thanked my host.

His lips spread into a suggestive grin. "Anything else?"

I told him, "No, thanks. I'll just..." I waved a hand toward the front door.

His turn to laugh.

Albert Burton's vitals were thus: Age seventy-seven; 182 pounds; hair—some; eyes—blue; address—106 Edgewater Street, Merlin Heights. Two of the days the private investigator spent on the Young/Burton case the injured man stayed home, but on the third day Albert and his wife, Ruth, set off on an adventure of errands that lasted three hours.

Armed with the PI's report, I started at the gas station where Ruth, who was driving, paid with a credit card. The attendant remembered absolutely nothing about the couple, which told me Al probably just sat there while Ruth signed for the gas.

Then on to the dry cleaner's—shirts, medium starch. Hubby waited in the car.

The dentist was another kettle of fish. Albert endured a long appointment in which he was fitted with a temporary crown.

Onward to the Bounce Back Physical Therapy Center where, according to the report, Al spent an hour and a quarter inside while Ruth went grocery shopping; the PI reported telltale bags being carried into their house.

Meanwhile, the building Albert had entered alone was a three-story Victorian painted an attractive dark blue/gray trimmed in white. Bounce Back occupied both sides of the first floor.

Over by the wall in the room to the left a patient tugged on yellow rubber tubing. "Exhale with exertion, Claire" the therapist advised before stepping behind a desk to greet me. Lithe and bubbly and blond as she was, I gauged that I could beat her in arm wrestling maybe four times out of five. No disrespect for the profession. I just lift more weights is all.

"Can you tell me whether Albert Burton kept his appointment on October twenty-ninth?" I inquired with a smile.

"Why do you ask?"

I explained that it was an insurance matter, and suddenly the therapist couldn't cooperate fast enough. Insurance money is our friend.

Yes, he had an appointment; and yes, he kept it, she told me.

"How's he coming along?"

"I don't think I'm supposed to..."

"There's quite a large dollar amount involved, Ms...." I checked her name plaque, "Kemp."

"Well, it does seem such a little thing...I guess I can tell you."

"Go ahead."

"He's made excellent progress."

"Oh?"

"Yes, his range of motion is almost back to normal."

"Excuse me?"

"His elbow. It's almost back to normal."

I could feel my lips pinch together. "Not my department," I remarked, finally releasing my breath. "Does anything about Albert Burton strike you as strange?"

She shrugged. "He's an old guy. They're all sort of strange."

"I mean was he all there...in the head."

"Whoa." The young woman actually backed off. "I'm not sure I..."

Why spook her over information she obviously wasn't willing to give? "You're right," I hastened to interrupt. Something about this exchange nagged at me though, something the therapist should have mentioned.

"Did anybody else come in to ask about Mr. Burton's appointment?"

Her face tilted with budding suspicion and mild surprise. "No."

I thanked her and retreated to the common center hall to decide what, if anything, that piece of information meant. That the private investigator was lazy? That he'd had to choose between staying out of sight and checking on something that appeared to be obvious?

While I was pondering, a door on the second floor opened and a couple in their fifties started down the stairs. The woman had a folder tucked under her arm, and both of their faces looked strained.

After they were gone, I went up to see what sort of office it was.

"Sorkin Financial Planners" read a discreet brass plaque affixed to the middle of the solid blue door. Probably another equally discreet one outside that I'd missed.

So most likely the departing couple had been discussing their assets with an expert in preparation for retirement. A few years ago, my father had sought such advice, and he'd come away with mixed feelings, possibly because he said his brain fried after about an hour of listening to the consultant talk.

What to do? What to do? There was a reason why a cop's badge is shaped like a shield. Without it, I would have to be soft-footed and sly, especially since I didn't even know whether Albert Burton was a client here.

The forty-something receptionist had dark hair cut fashionably short, a mauve manicure and a lavender suit. The suit jacket hung on a brass clothes tree back in the corner.

"Good morning," a glance at her watch, "or is it afternoon?"

"Whatever you say," I told her affably.

Her lips tried a smile before puzzlement overruled. Obviously, I lacked the years and worried aspect of their typical client; and even if I did have an appointment, it was lunchtime and that made me at least an hour early.

"I'm hoping you can help me," I began.

"I'll try."

"Has Uncle Burt been in here bothering you?"

"That would be Burt...?"

"Oh, sorry. Albert Burton. Somebody told my mother he stopped in here while Ruth went to the grocery store. Maybe last Tuesday?"

"Yes. Mr. Burton came in, but I wouldn't say he was bothering us. He had an appointment with Mr. Smith."

My heart did a little giddy up. "Oh, dear," I lamented, staring off into space and chewing my lip.

"What's the matter?" she asked.

"It's just that...this is so delicate." I pretended to effect scruples. "It's just that the family is talking about having Uncle Burt declared incompetent. I don't think he is, but some of the others, well, most of the others..."

A man materialized in the doorway, probably the esteemed Mr. Smith. "Nonsense," he said. An educated type with spectacles and thinning hair, he wore shirtsleeves and a loosened club tie. "I've been working with Mr. Burton for weeks, and I don't mind telling you the man is sharp as a tack."

My senses were now keened up to the max. The trick was to hide my excitement behind make-believe doubt. "Really? He remembers your name and everything?"

"Of course."

"How about trusts and IRAs and variable annuities? Does he understand all of those, because a lot of the family thinks he's, shall we say...lost his edge?"

The investment advisor dug in behind his folded arms. "No one who has worked with him as I have would say that."

"Oh, wonderful. What a relief." I clamped my hands together with hearty self-congratulation. "Now there's just one more thing."

"What?"

"How about putting that in writing. Just a sentence or two. Something to show the family..."

"I don't think..."

"... and the lawyers. You know what sticklers they can be."

Instinctively I'd straightened my back, and the change of posture may have made Smith smell a rat. "What is this?" he demanded.

"You first. Will you sign a statement saying that Albert Burton is still capable of handling his own assets?"

Smith's consternation clearly conveyed how he felt about interfering relatives. "Oh, all right," he conceded, "but only to help Mr. Burton retain control."

"It never hurts to tell the truth," a remark that would haunt me before the day's end.

After a panicked glance at her boss, Lavender Suit allowed me to borrow her computer, and in a few minutes I had both her signature and her boss's on a printout affirming that, in their opinion, Albert Burton was completely fit to conduct his own business affairs.

"I thank you," I told them both, "and the Amalgamated Insurance Association of North America thanks you, too."

When you've been out of touch for more than four years, getting beeped by your boss is a startling and exhilarating experience. It happened just as I sped past the Willow Grove exit of the Pennsylvania turnpike, so I steered into the first emergency pull-off and punched David's number into my personal cell phone with trembling fingers. I was so full of myself for solving Bob Battersby's case that I actually expected to be congratulated on my victory.

Instead, David said, "Please stop by the office at your earliest possible convenience."

Okay, so he hadn't heard the news yet—how could he have? I would tell him myself when I got there.

Forty minutes later I stepped into the SIU portion of the claims domain still flushed with pride and kiting on adrenaline. David's door was open. I tapped on the doorjamb to announce my presence.

"Come in, come in," the SIU supervisor suggested, lines of concern between his fair eyebrows.

Draped across the nearest chair, Bob Battersby preened one of those hideous hook-shaped sideburns with an index finger. Rather than sidle past the other investigator again, I stood beside him and tried to look at ease.

David was also standing, so we were more or less eye to eye. Yellow shirtsleeves rolled up, hair tumbling onto his forehead, his hands were so fidgety that he had to clamp them under his arms.

"I just got a disturbing call from a Mr. Peter Smith," he finally remarked. "He's a financial advisor with Sorkin..."

"I know who he is."

"Oh," David said as if he had expected a denial. "Then you admit you were there."

"Yes. I asked about Albert Burton's mental state. Smith swore the old guy is still sharp as a tack, and so did his assistant. They both signed a statement."

"I see. Well, Mr. Smith took exception to the method you used to extract that information from him and Ms. Loffland. You can't go around lying to people, Lauren. It isn't ethical."

So that was it. "One little fib," I argued, "that just happened to save the company two million dollars. It isn't illegal—cops do it all the time."

"One point six," David corrected me. "Burton had hospital expenses due to the injury." He experimented with a smile. "So yes, ethics aside, you did good."

Suddenly, Bob became a sideshow. Red-faced, he popped upright in his chair and pressed his palms against the edge of David's desk. "That's it?" he fumed. "That's all you're going to say?"

David gripped his hands behind his backside and smiled a little wider.

Gaping with disbelief, Bob glared at David for a couple of beats then bulled past me out the door, the fury in his eyes like a shadow across my grave. Welcome to Corporate America.

Now the Little League field lies far behind me, home a mere two blocks ahead. As I gradually slow my pace to a cooling walk, I shudder to think how Bob had hiked himself right up to the District Manager to report my heinous lie "for the sake of the company." If David hadn't intervened, I'd have lost my job, an outcome that would have benefitted Bob not one whit but would have landed me in serious financial trouble.

Tired, wet with sweat, still confused by Battersby's behavior, I let myself back into the still-empty house. Why had he risked going behind David's back about something that I didn't dare do again, even if it had worked in the company's favor? Was he that much of a prick? Was I that much of a threat? It seemed so extreme, so senseless. I just didn't get it. But one thing I knew. Someone with that much anger just might pick up a phone to fill a mourning daughter's head with suspicion.

Apparently I needed to know a lot more about Bob Battersby.

And I needed to know it soon.

Chapter 5

I've just guzzled two glasses of water at the kitchen sink and grabbed a handful of stale pretzel sticks. I'm not sure if family typically leaves a funeral reception first or last, but one thing is certain—Nina won't want to see me anymore than I want to see her.

On my way upstairs I'm drawn to the doorway of Corinne's bedroom. Perhaps it's the accumulated hours she spent in this space, or my imagination combined with my need, but I sense my late friend's presence here more than I did at the church. With her quilted brocade bedspread glowing in the waning light, I can't resist. I curl up on it like a child in a mother's lap—pretzel crumbs and all.

With memories of Corinne's final hours consuming me, my tears finally fall.

SOAMES MEMORIAL only doles out two passes per hour per patient, so just getting into the Intensive Care Unit to see Corinne had been difficult. Nina had first dibs, of course, but even though I was the only one asking, the brunette biddy on duty refused me on the grounds that I wasn't immediate family.

Knowing they could break their own rules anytime they suspected a patient might be dying, I requested that she ask Corinne's doctor to make an exception. During one of my worst complications hadn't they almost let Brent in before my father told them absolutely no?

The volunteer's spine stiffened, but she did reach for the phone.

With obvious reluctance she began to tell the doctor I was, "almost a relative…"

"Oh, hell, give me that." I lifted the receiver out of her hand.

"Who is this?" a cultured male voice demanded.

"Lauren Beck. I live with Corinne Wilder. And you would be…?"

"Dr. Joshua Brooks. Are you saying you live in Mrs. Wilder's house?"

"Yes. She nursed me through Hodgkins when she was dating my father, and I've been helping with her relapse, *was* helping, until her daughter moved in last weekend."

"I see," he mused, then paused long enough for me to worry that he'd heard about my outburst in the hall outside the hospital pharmacy. Nina had dropped her mother's latest CEA count on me like the Hiroshima bomb, and in my panic I said some pretty irresponsible things to one of the nurses about Corinne's chemotherapy.

Dr. Brooks told me to put the receptionist back on the line.

"Okay, sure," I agreed, "but do you mind if I ask why?" If he intended to refuse my request, I wanted another chance to argue.

"I was going to tell her to give you the pass. Isn't that what you want?"

"Yes," I said. "Yes! But there's something else you need to know." If Nina reacted to my arrival the way I expected, Brooks should probably be forewarned, especially if I ever hoped to visit again.

"Her daughter dislikes me because, because she's…" *jealous* sounded too self serving, so I mumbled something about Nina being an only child.

The doctor took a moment to think. Then he reminded me that the ICU admits visitors around the clock.

"Oh?" I remarked, but then I caught on. "Good idea. *Great* idea. Thanks, Doc. Thank you very much."

"Now may I speak to the receptionist?" he asked, and this time I relinquished the phone.

After Dr. Brooks gave the receptionist permission for me to visit, I left the hospital, drove to a nearby diner, and lingered over coffee as long as I could. Then I laid low in the hospital parking lot until Nina finally emerged from her vigil. The taillights of her Subaru weren't yet out of sight before I rushed inside to collect my yellow plastic visitor's pass.

At night the Intensive Care Unit's lighting was dimmed and the bustle subdued. Even the beeps of the monitors seemed quieter. Some patients were still receiving animated attention but most were asleep in their curtained cubicles.

From the shift nurse assigned to Corinne I learned that a chest x-ray had revealed bilateral infiltrates, in other words congestion in both lungs, or pneumonia. She was also spiking a fever, and in between deep wrenching coughs her respirations were shallow and quick, perhaps thirty-five to forty a minute. Factor in Corinne's precariously low white cell count and you've got a woman in serious danger.

I thanked the nurse then approached Corinne's partition with careful footsteps. The low light of the monitors revealed that she'd been dressed in a blue hospital gown with a thin robe for warmth. Her frazzled gray-brown hair fanned out across the pillow, and her eyelids twitched with troubled dreams. In spite of the oxygen she was receiving through nasal prongs, each wet, shallow breath underscored how precious time with her had become.

For most of my allotted ten minutes I watched her sleep. When her eyes suddenly blinked open, I reached over to brush the hair from her brow.

She turned toward me with surprise. "What time?" she asked.

"Ten-thirty," I answered. So much to say, nowhere to begin. I settled for stroking her hand.

"Nina?"

"She went home. How do you feel?"

"Shitty." Slurred, but heartfelt.

"The antibiotic hasn't had time to work," I remarked, and Corinne grunted her opinion of that.

I'd been issued a face mask to protect her from anything I might be carrying, and I began to worry that she couldn't see how much I loved her. And no, I couldn't just say the words. If it came off sounding too sentimental, Corinne would think I thought she was dying. Then she might think so, too.

"Nina," she repeated, and the way her face was etched with concern I wondered whether the drugs had confused her, whether she thought I was her natural daughter.

Then she touched my arm and murmured, "Sorry," and I realized she was worried about me and her daughter living under the same roof. "Nina," she whispered between breaths, "Nina...needed..."

"It's okay," I assured her. "She loves you dearly, and right now she should have as much time with you as she can get. Don't worry about it. I understand."

"Mind?"

"No, I don't mind either. It's a chance for her and me to get better acquainted." So far not a joy either way, but a true statement nonetheless. I did believe Nina needed to be with her mother as much as possible. Then if the worst actually came to pass, she would know she had done everything a daughter possibly could.

Too soon a shadow appeared at the opening of the curtain, the nurse politely reminding me my time was up. I waved a hand to acknowledge the hint, and the woman turned away. She wouldn't forget about me though, so I really did need to leave.

I stood up and removed my mask. Then I kissed my fingers and touched them to Corinne's cheek. Her coal black eyes locked onto mine, and for a moment I convinced myself that she was as hungry for my affection as I was for hers.

"Love you," I said, ignoring my own advice.

Corinne nodded once then averted her eyes.

I tore myself away.

When I emerged from the hospital, I encountered a night mist so thick and cold it might as well have been rain. Underdressed for the chill, I hustled out to the Miata and started up the engine.

Behind me another vehicle instantly came alive, and the coincidence unnerved me. I had sensed no other movements in the parking lot, heard no footsteps other than mine. So the driver must have been waiting inside his vehicle. A van maybe, or a pickup? The headlight beams shone level with my shoulders.

I put my car in motion, and the other vehicle began to follow.

Maybe Jimmy Tanner, one of the fraud cases I was investigating? Ridiculous. Probably just another late visitor who had taken some time to collect himself. I could certainly identify with that.

Except normal visiting hours were long over, and I'd been the last outsider to leave the ICU.

Then an employee just waking up from a catnap. I refused to be spooked by the late hour, the weather, the stress of Corinne's new problem.

I turned right out of the back driveway, and when the truck or van or whatever it was slid back out of view, I devoted my attention to the road.

Landis, our small city, becomes a small town at night. Stop lights are tokens, as useful as the traffic controls on a Lionel landscape in somebody's basement. As soon as I could, I rolled into a right turn as if I were the only driver around.

Except I wasn't. The dark pickup—I'd gotten that much from my rearview mirror—was still with me. After ten minutes and two turns, I humored my nerves and drove around the block until I was headed back in the same direction, the direction I needed to get home.

The pickup followed, looking almost casual back there, as if the driver was some guy playing around. It happens. Forgetting that women get raped by sickos all the time, a dumb yutz decides to stick to my tail like a rude old dog. What a shock they get when I double back and grab them by the throat.

Tonight I was too worn down to bother. When I hit a straightaway outside of town, I floored it.

A country mile before Corinne's street I nosed the Miata into a condo complex, slipped into a parking spot facing the road, killed the engine and the lights. My service piece was back home, but I kept a can of mace in the glove compartment for backup. That and some common sense would have to do.

In less than a minute the pickup chugged by going ten miles an hour. The driver was shadowed, of course, so I couldn't tell whether he was hunting for me or if he'd already caught sight of the Miata and was thumbing his nose. Regardless, he sped up before I could read more than the first three letters of his license plate. GRS something.

I watched until the truck's taillights disappeared. After a prudent pause, I headed home with the mace by my side.

At nine forty-five the next morning the perky Information volunteer handing me my visitor's pass answered, "Yes, Dr. Brooks is on this weekend." When I asked what he looked like, she held her hand at collar-bone level and stage whispered that he wore rimless glasses and was "bald on top."

I kept a lookout for white coats, and just as I reached the Intensive Care Unit the wide double doors parted and a shy man fitting the volunteer's description emerged.

"Hello," I said, stepping into his path. "I'm Lauren Beck, Corinne Wilder's, um, close friend. I think we spoke on the phone yesterday."

"Yes?"

I fanned myself with the yellow ICU pass. "I'd like to hug you for this, but I see that you're wearing a wedding band."

The little guy actually blushed and lowered his eyes. "No problem. Now, if you don't mind...?" He glanced longingly toward the nearby snack shop.

"Please. Just tell me Corinne's prognosis—the real one."

A double-take and, finally, a spark of rapport. "Now I remember. You had..."

"Hodgkin's, yes."

Brooks's face warmed with empathy—he was speaking to a survivor.

Scanning the floor, he waved his head. "Your friend is..." A sense of motion behind me. "Oh, Ms. Wilder. Good morning." A new blush ignited the physician's ears and spread upward beyond his former hairline. "I was just about to tell Ms. Beck that we're giving your mother a second antibiotic. Also, I've taken the precaution of asking an infectious disease specialist to look in on her."

I stepped back until the doctor and Corinne's daughter were closer to each other than to me, but it wasn't enough subservience to suit Nina. Her shoulders hunched and her chin lifted.

One glance between us and Brooks drew her farther away. "Let's give Ms. Beck a moment with your mother while we..."

"But..." Nina protested as Brooks guided her farther down the hall.

"Only a moment or two and then you'll have your whole ten minutes. We need to talk over a few things. It's Nina isn't it?"

"Yes, but..."

The doctor's eyes signaled for me to get a move on.

Corinne's curtained cubicle was the fourth one in on the right. She was awake, sitting up, and receiving oxygen through something I've heard called a ventimask, most likely because the nasal prongs weren't effective enough. Her eyes darted like sparrows, and her hands couldn't keep still.

"How's it going?" I asked.

She glanced my way briefly then resumed her anxious quest for air.

The curtain parted, and Nina was on me like a banshee.

"Get out," she shouted, causing the whole unit to gasp.

I should have retreated, but I was too stunned to move. Stares prickled my skin, and I didn't trust myself to speak.

Making elaborate shushing motions as he rushed toward us, Dr. Brooks addressed Nina. "Okay, okay," he told her. "There she is." He ushered Corinne's daughter into the cubicle then forcefully steered me out.

He didn't let go until we reached the hall. Then he put his hands on his hips and waved his head. "What are we going to do with you?" he seemed to ask the floor.

Panic was just a word away. He could not, *could not* kick me out.

"Listen," I said, before he launched into a serious scold. "How about if I lay low until you tell me I can go back in? And if Nina starts up like that again, I promise I'll run for the exit."

"No. I don't think..."

"Please! I'll be good. I'll be an angel."

"You're not..."

"...a relative. I know." The admission vacuumed every last bit of spunk from my body. The doctor had to grab my arm again, this time to steady me.

I held my breath, and he finally relented. "You'll leave at the first sign of trouble?"

"I swear."

11:55 a.m.

For the long intervals between visits Nina had taken the non-denominational chapel close to the ICU for her own, which was fine with me. I got the waiting room and all its perks—free coffee, magazines, and a vending machine. I needed all the distractions I could get.

By eleven-thirty I'd already read or rejected most of the magazines and had taken to paranoid speculations about the truck that followed me home the previous night, an anomaly I couldn't seem to leave alone. When I started imagining the driver as Brent W. Cahill, which was beyond absurd, I decided it was time to get up and move around. Anything to keep from dwelling on Corinne's condition.

I was exiting the rest room when I heard Nina imploring one of the ICU nurses. "...but it's her grandmother. I don't understand why she can't come."

"Absolutely not," the nurse maintained. "Against the rules. Now if you'll excuse me..." She ducked her head and plodded off.

Too self-involved to notice me, Nina huffed over to punch the wall switch for the double doors. As soon as she could slip through the opening, she power walked into the ICU. In ten minutes, with luck, I would get another turn of my own. Meanwhile, I would indulge myself and peek through the window.

Nina had come to a halt in front of her mother's cubicle. Now she parted the curtains to glance inside. She dropped her purse. She shouted something. Hands swinging like a marionette's, she shouted again. And again. A male nurse rushed to respond, followed by a female and finally Dr. Brooks.

I couldn't tear my eyes away.

Nina retrieved her purse. Clutching it to her chest she ran toward the exit where I stood. The doors parted, and I looked into glazed eyes that recognized nothing. A whimper of fear, and Nina was gone.

I was inside before the doors swung shut.

Crazed by oxygen deprivation, Corinne had ripped off her ventimask. She was leaning over her bedside table, almost crawling over it in an effort to climb out of bed. Her eyes were wide, her lips rimmed in blue, her hair and gown soaked with perspiration. Dr. Brooks and an orderly were trying to keep her in bed, but their efforts failed. Orders were shouted, and a nurse almost bowled me down in her rush to obey.

I backed out and stumbled past the chapel, scarcely hearing Nina's sobs over the buzz in my head.

The agony Corinne was enduring defied all that was fair and logical, and I couldn't deal with that. My whole being begged for somewhere to lay the blame.

Before I knew it I was getting off the elevator at the second floor, propelling myself like a B-movie zombie toward the chemotherapy suite. Yet even before the person at the sign-in desk informed me that my former nurse, Amy Dion, had the day off, I recognized myself as a pathetic, desperate woman grasping at straws. Chastened, I turned back into the hall, where the same in-house pharmacist who'd overheard my previous outburst was working behind the dispensary window.

I hesitated, but not for long.

"Excuse me," I interrupted. "Could you please answer a question?"

Her "yes" was curt, bordering on rude. She remembered me.

"I'm wondering if you can tell me how you go about preparing the chemotherapy IVs."

A further stiffening of her back, hostility in her whole bearing. She had seen through my careful wording and took offense at the implication.

"Not my job," she said. "Now why don't you mind your own business and let me get back to work?"

I'd insulted her. A complete stranger.

Retreating to the elevator bank, I heard the pharmacist's words as a warning: Get a grip on yourself, girl—and do it now.

4:35 p.m.

Corinne's acute respiratory distress had been resolved with sedation and a ventilator, if knocking out someone unable to process enough oxygen can be said to resolve anything. I couldn't help visualizing her face covered with a pillow, her arms flailing...but that was just a momentary nightmare, the punctuation of a very long afternoon.

I caught up with Dr. Brooks just after he finished with a patient. He seemed eager for me to follow Nina's example and go home.

"How is she?" I inquired. Last time he had reported that three antibiotics and white cell stimulators had failed to improve Corinne's blood count.

"Too soon to say," he recited with a weak smile. A deflection, but a forgivable one. If the news was good, I wouldn't have had to ask.

"One more minute with her and then I'll go, too."

He nodded, but his mind had already moved on.

I parted the curtain and slipped inside the dimly lit compartment with Corinne. Everything around her was again clean and tidy, proffering the impression of promise and peace, an illusion I'd had all afternoon to see through. Nina, unfortunately, still clung to the fiction as if it were scripture. I pitied her; she would be facing reality unprepared, and probably all too soon.

This time I stood at the end of Corinne's bed, viewing her from a sort of middle distance. Her struggle, if it could still be called that, seemed token if not already lost. Still, I trusted that she could sense my presence the way I'd sensed hers when our roles had been reversed.

The notion was folly, of course. Anyone sedated enough to tolerate a tube down her throat was past knowing whether anyone was nearby.

I squeezed Corinne's foot through the blanket. Then I left.

7:49 p.m.

Nina had been out when I got home. Now she burst into Corinne's unlighted kitchen complaining loudly to herself, "The zoo. The ZOO!" She flipped a switch, brightening the living room to a painful degree.

"What?" I croaked from my corner of the brown chintz sofa. Bobble heads and cookie jars stared back at me like Halloween goblins.

"Lauren!" she gasped. "What are you doing down here?"

"I'm coping." My date with Jose Cuervo had begun during the drive home from the hospital and progressed so hot and heavy that we hadn't quite found our way upstairs to bed. Soon, though. The pint bottle I'd bought was nearly gone. "And you?"

Nina responded with a manic eagerness that I trusted the way an abused wife trusts men. "I wanted to bring Jilly back with me," she finished pouring a glass of wine then brandished it like a stage prop, "but Todd, the bastard, is taking her to the zoo tomorrow. The zoo! His head is so far up his butt..." She left the thought unfinished. Switched abruptly to her mother.

"Did you see her?" she enthused. "She looks so much better, don't you think?"

Even with my mind totally blurred by tequila, I knew better than to reply. I lifted myself off the sofa and stumbled out of the room.

9:42 a.m., Sunday

My eyelids were made of sandpaper, and my clothes didn't feel like my clothes. Head throbbing, I drove back to the Landis diner and forced down three aspirins with my two-egg breakfast. Today I would use the hospital's valet service. I was in no condition to save money.

Dr. Brooks nodded to me from the near side of the nurses' station. His look of hard wear was still in place, only the shave and shirt were new. "Where's the other one?" he wondered.

"Church. I'm going to take off after this." I handed him my cell phone number on a slip of paper and asked him to use it if anything happened.

He gave me a questioning look but stuffed the paper into his pocket. Why quarrel with a decision that would only make his day easier?

This morning Corinne's lips moved almost imperceptibly, like someone concentrating hard on reading a book. Otherwise, she was sleeping so deeply she scarcely seemed animate. I stroked her hair, held her hand. Ten minutes passed by like nothing.

As I kissed her good-bye, tears I'd been unaware of slipped onto her cheek.

"Love you," I whispered one last time.

When my cell phone rang, I was on Route 422 racing toward Lancaster county at seventy miles an hour. I didn't answer; and, mercifully, Dr. Brooks left no message.

The kitchen door clunks shut, and I awaken with a start. I am still on Corinne's bed, my hair dry and my body cold. Judging by the darkness, I slept at least an hour.

Whatever Nina is doing downstairs sounds careless and angry. She's seen both my company car and the Miata; she knows I'm here.

I don't want to get caught in Corinne's room, but I've crushed some of the pretzels. Hastily sweeping them into my hand, I turn—and gasp. Nina is standing in the doorway.

"Get out," she shrieks even more venomously than before. "Out of this room and out of this house."

"Right now?"

"Yes! Don't make me call the police."

I wave my head, disheartened but not surprised. Hating me seems to be the only relief the woman can fabricate for herself, and she is nowhere near ready to let it go.

"You'll have to return some of my rent," I tell her, marveling that I've managed to keep my voice even, "and my food money." I'm not due a paycheck yet, and I would rather not starve just to make Nina happy.

Her eyes pop open then abruptly narrow.

"I'll put some money on the kitchen counter," she announces. "Pick it up on your way out."

Chapter 6

After Nina's eviction notice, I hurry upstairs to pack some stuff.

"Hey," I greet my roommate with phony cheer. "Looks like we're outta here."

No response except for the bubble machine, but none of my goldfish have been much for words, a good reason to love them, in my opinion.

As usual, my whitewashed attic aerie is a mess of floral-cushioned wicker chairs draped with laundry. A decent computer/printer setup fills one window alcove, a dusty old TV resides in another. Wind whistles through the loose old sashes in winter and causes me to wear a bathrobe and a wool hat to bed. The iron bedstead came out of my dad's barn and complements the wicker set whenever I tidy up; but, to be honest, cleaning fell off my priority list back when I was sick and has yet to make a comeback.

I've loved holing up here away from the world, but Corinne was right. It's time for me to move on. I dig my duffel out of the corner and begin to fill it with whatever comes to hand.

I'm gathering things from the bathroom when I sense a presence in the attic doorway–Jilly, wearing her good funeral clothes and a very vulnerable, very perplexed expression. If I crossed the room to give her a hug, would she run?

"You heard," I state instead. Everybody witnessed her mother's outburst at the church annex, and nobody within fifty feet of the house missed the ultimatum Nina delivered only moments ago.

"I haven't done anything," I tell the little girl carefully. "I loved your grandmother."

Jilly shrugs as if it doesn't matter, but her lips are trembling.

I drop a handful of cosmetics into my duffel bag and ease a little closer. "Actually, I'm glad you're here," I tell her. "I wanted to see you before I go, but I also need to ask a favor."

"What?" She's still distrustful, still ready to bolt.

"Think you can take care of my goldfish?" It was a snap decision, but a good one. I have no idea where I'm going.

Jilly glances toward the bubbling, lighted tank on the dresser and Swimmie stares back, a little desperately, I think.

"Of course, if it would get you in trouble with your mother..."

The girl shoots me the same conspirator's eyes she did the night I dropped her off at her father's. "My mother doesn't know everything I do."

"I guess not," I agree, feeling better about this kid by the minute.

"His name is Swimmie," I tell her. "My mom won him for me at a church fair when I was five." The original one, I might have mentioned; this was Swimmie Number Six or Seven.

Jilly's nose crinkles, indicating that the name is too juvenile for her eight-year-old sensibilities.

"...but you can call him whatever you want," I concede.

"Cousteau," she announces with a decisive nod, and the deal is sealed.

I recognize a little jab of jealousy, or maybe regret. "I'll pick him up when I come back for the rest of my stuff," I tell Jilly. Best to be up front about that.

"Whatever." Again with the phony disinterest.

I slip the kid a few dollars for fish food and am about to describe how to keep my scaly friend alive when we hear Nina's voice.

"Gotta go." Jilly runs for the door.

"Wait! You don't know how to..."

"Internet," the kid replies as she bounds down the stairs.

I forgot that even eight-year-olds know how to look up things online.

While I finish packing, I tell Swimmie guilty things like, "Don't worry," and, "It'll be alright," and especially, "I'll be back for you." Then I sling the duffel over my shoulder and grab my purse. The last thing I say over the lump in my throat is, "Sorry, little guy. I'll miss you."

And everything about my life in this place.

I take the Taurus, figuring that I'll return for my personal vehicle over the weekend. First stop, the diner near the hospital that offers plenty of good, cheap food.

Waiting for a mouthful of black beans and rice to cool, it occurs to me that I should have left Nina a note. "Pick up the rest asap." Something like that. I have visions of the Miata with four flat tires and "KILLER" scratched in the paint, my other belongings strewn all over the yard or on the curb along with the trash.

"Damn," I say out loud, which draws a sharp glance from my server. With a world-weary sigh I tell her I broke up with my boyfriend, a quicker explanation than the truth.

She rolls her blue eyes and shakes her blonde head, drops off a platter of meatloaf, then touches the back of my shoulder. "Been there, Sweetie," she commiserates. "Getcha anything else?"

"Just the check."

Since my credit-card limit isn't enormous and some of it has already been used, I pay for my meal with ten bucks of Nina's cash. The tip is too little, but it's the best I can do.

Over the weekend I'll hunt for an apartment, but until then it might as well be the Lucky Leaf Motel outside of Landis. Both cheap and convenient, it has two rectangular strips of rooms with a quaint white clapboard office in between. Cable TV is advertised just above the red neon "Vacancy" sign. Everything a homeless woman can possibly want.

The tiny registration area smells of mold, and there is no place to sit.

"Hep ya?" the night man inquires, scrutinizing me openly. Tall and balding, his skeptical expression appears to be permanent.

"A room please. Non-smoking."

The man grabs a key from the row of mailboxes on the wall and slaps it on the counter. "How many nights?"

"Two." The price is fair but nothing I want to pay for long.

"In advance." His smile is more smirk than leer, so I figure he pegs me as a runaway wife, the reason I brought my duffel in with me. No luggage tells another story altogether.

The clerk slides my VISA card through his machine, reads the message, and hits cancel. Slides it through again, then puts it in his shirt pocket.

"Hey!"

"Sorry, Miss. Company says to confiscate yer card."

"Try it again."

"No can do."

Wouldn't you just know. "There has to be some mistake."

"Nope. No mistake."

Okay, Lauren, deal with that tomorrow. Right now you need a place to sleep.

"How about I write you a check?" Until I find out what happened to my credit, I'm afraid to part with any more cash.

"Not on yer life." His lips flick in and out of a smile. Then suddenly he's leaning across the counter close enough to touch my arm.

"Might be we could work out a deal, eh? Trade favors, so to speak. Whutdaya say?" Same old same old.

"Thanks, but no thanks," I tell him as I back toward the door.

I throw the duffle in the trunk of the Taurus and climb behind the wheel. Tell myself no big deal. Phone somebody. Bum a night on a sofa. Figure out what's what in the morning.

The problem is who to call. As Corinne frequently reminded me, all my other friendships died from neglect.

Garry from the bar? At least I saw him within recent memory. He even shouted for me to get the hell over there and give him a kiss.

Garry from the bar. Adores his wife, and everybody knows it. So maybe she trusts him enough to believe that I'm no threat to her marriage, that I'm really and truly stuck and only want to borrow their sofa for one night.

I dig my cell phone out of my shoulder bag and punch in 4-1-1. Yet instead of the musical beeps that precede the "What city and state?" question, I get a terse robotic message.

"Service has been temporarily suspended..."

Chapter 7

Dumbfounded, I sit in the Taurus outside the Lucky Leaf Motel marveling at how perfectly someone screwed up my life.

And how stupid I've been. Maybe, just maybe, if Corinne hadn't been ill, I would have picked up the warning signs in time—the truck that followed me from the hospital, the opened mail. But then again, maybe not. Who expects to be the recipient of so much spite?

Damn. No credit card. No phone. Thanks to Nina's crazy accusation, no place to live. A genuine pain in the ass situation, but in the great scheme of things still just a pea under my mattress, future cocktail conversation. "Once upon a time I actually had to..."

To what? I'd rather sleep in my car than go back to Corinne's—pardon me—*Nina's* house. For all I know she's the one behind all this.

Just to be moving, I nose the car up to the highway, look right then left.

Forget the crack about Nina, sleeping in the Taurus is not an option. Cars have locks that can be picked and transparent windows that can be smashed. Until I know who has it in for me, I want walls. Food and running water would be nice, too.

I time my entry into traffic and step on the gas.

Soon I'm leaving civilization behind—too far behind—so I make a hasty turn into a haven of streetlights and brick buildings, slow to a casual cruise that allows me to think...

Note to self: Reinstate my cell service first thing tomorrow.

No, scratch that—and not just because the idea of using a violated cell phone gives me the creeps. Somebody who hates me has my number, billing code, the works. I'm not sure what they can do with the information beside what they've already done, but leaving my phone turned off for now seems safest.

Five more minutes of driving aimlessly and biting my lip yields one possible host for the night, although it's already nine and he probably goes to bed early. Still, I'm short on ideas; so I head for Norman Schmidt's.

Dad's old friend lives in a three-bedroom brick cottage of the white-picket-fence variety. The surrounding neighborhood is dotted with others just like it along with a few that have been expanded to accommodate children or hobbies. The developer named his project Glendenning Village, but it used to be the Heckler farm. Dad brokered it soon after Clive Heckler's boy died in a helicopter accident. Last I heard Heckler Senior lives in Ft. Lauderdale, his mind so gone that he might as well be living in Timbuktu. Not my day for cheery thoughts.

I park in Norman's short driveway and approach the front door.

No answer to my polite tap, so I pound a little harder, and in a few minutes Dad's old buddy finally opens the door. His jug-handle ears are silhouetted by the hall light, his eyebrows hiding under a forelock of curly gray hair. I notice that his blue and white plaid bathrobe is untied, revealing striped pajamas that aren't buttoned quite right.

"Lauren!" he greets me. "What are you doing here?"

He gestures me inside; and as I ease past, I notice alcohol on his breath. His eyes are red-rimmed, too.

"It was the funeral," he remarks as if I've said something. "Sally..." he waves his hand in an all-encompassing circle. "It reminded me of Sally."

I realize now that he's been crying, and I can't resist throwing my arms around him. Then I remember the open bathrobe and quickly let go.

"I understand," I say. "I do. And I'm very sorry to intrude, but I'm really in trouble. It's sort of a long story, but I don't have anywhere to sleep tonight."

"Nina." Norman nods, delicately referencing this afternoon's scene while staring at his feet.

When the moment begins to drag, I bend down to catch his eye. "Norman? Is it okay if I stay?"

He blinks and answers, "Of course, Jellybean," but his hands hop and drop helplessly. "What exactly do you need?"

"You got a guest room? If not, a sofa and a blanket would be fine. I'm pretty low maintenance."

"The upstairs is...well, not ready for company. You sure the sofa will be okay?"

"Uncle Norm, tonight your floor would feel like a featherbed."

"You can use the upstairs bathroom to wash up, but the other rooms..."

"That's just terrific. Honest." I cup his chin with my fingers and kiss his cheek. "Just one more thing," I add. "You got any more of that stuff you've been drinking?"

His round elf face suddenly beams. "Long Island iced tea," which, if I recall correctly, is roughly the proof of antifreeze. "You really want some?"

"No, I really want a lot."

Norman's kitchen is small and dated, with blue Formica counters and a faux-brick backsplash. The window over the sink has a ruffled white café curtain adorned with cobwebs and grease. No microwave, just a white porcelain gas stove with black burner grids. Sally hasn't been with us for quite some time.

The first few sips of the tall, icy drink Norman sets in front of me melts away some of the chill I've been feeling. I'm so relieved and grateful and tired that I'm surprised I can keep my head up. But then, elbows splayed on the table, we begin to dredge up mutual memories, pleasant ones from before Dad sold the farm to finance my recovery and his retirement, before he baffled and saddened both of us by moving away.

"How about that smell you got soon as soon as you walked into Tom's hardware store?" Norm challenges. "Whatdya think that was?"

I laugh as I try to guess. "Old diapers? Paint thinner? Tom?"

Norm waves his head, tells me a part-timer spilled a gallon of rancid linseed oil near the heat vent. "Never could get rid of the stink."

"Sorta like my dad's cooking," I decide.

Norman's head slips lower on his fist. "Didn't he have a pet duck for a while?"

I roll my eyes. "Yeah, a male mallard." It limped when it walked making it a bona fide lame duck, so Dad named him Congress. "Nasty bird," I recall. "Bit me in the bum and left a scar."

"Show you mine, if you show me yours," Norman slurs.

I give that a crooked smile. Then I get up to pour myself another. I wave a bottle in Norman's direction, but he pushes his tumbler away. "Off to bed," he says. "Make yerself at home."

Before he shambles off I ask permission to borrow his phone. "Long distance?" It's time to acknowledge the second heartache of my day, the fact that my father didn't come back east for the funeral.

Norman tosses a hand. "Knock yerself out," he answers. "I got unlimited."

Slumped on the sofa next to the phone, I arrange my thoughts as Norman goes through his bedtime routine on the floor above. When at last I feel as ready as I'm ever going to, I lift the receiver and dial. Albuquerque is in an earlier time zone; I won't be waking anybody up.

The wrong voice says, "Hello?" but I do my best to sound cordial.

"Annie, it's me, Lauren," I tell my new step-mother. "Is dad around?"

"Of course, honey. I'll get him. Charlie, Charlie, *phone*. It's your daughter." Her southern accent sounds so cheerful I'm almost convinced that whatever makes Dad happy makes her happy, too.

Then an unwelcome thought intrudes. Did my devotion to Corinne warp my attitude toward this woman? Possibly. But then Dad gets on the line, and hurt crowds out all reason.

"The funeral was today," I remark, and the implied *Where were you?* isn't lost on my father. His silence lasts about as long it takes to recover from a surprise punch.

He sighs before he says, "She didn't want me there, Beanie."

I try not to gasp. "You two talked about that?"

"We did."

"Before you left?" In a day of shocking events this is one jolt too many. I can't seem to stop blinking.

"No," he says in the patient manner that isn't patient at all. "Last week. Corinne didn't tell you?" Another sigh, as if he's tired of being judged by me, tired of being misunderstood.

"I'm sorry, Dad. Start at the beginning. It's been a long day."

So he does. He tells me he and Corinne spoke about once a month since he moved to New Mexico and that during their last conversation–scarcely eight days ago–she told him to stay home if and when. "Don't waste your money, she said. Just put on some music and raise a glass to old times."

This is something I should easily accept, so why do I still feel trapped under a truck?

Because I wanted him and Corinne to warm their stockinged feet by the fire, sip cocoa with marshmallows and gossip about their friends. I wanted holidays at the old homestead with Ron's kids running roughshod through the house. Corinne would bake ziti and buy pumpkin pies and Dad would serve his disgusting mulled wine. I wanted a whole family, especially since chemo had ruined any chance of creating one for myself.

Then there's also the other thing, the one I don't like to admit. Dad didn't just leave Corinne behind; he left me behind, too.

"So did you?" I all but challenge.

"Did I what?"

"Listen to music and toast Corinne?"

"Not yet, Beanie. But I will. I will."

I only met Annie briefly the weekend of their wedding, so I can't gauge how she might react to her husband toasting the memory of another woman. For her sake I let this one slide, but it isn't easy.

"So how are you?" Dad asks.

I pause before I answer. "I've been better," I reply, "but I guess I've been worse."

When he says, "I hear you, Beanie. I hear you," I know we're both thinking of the times I almost died myself.

"Love you, Dad." I tell him, meaning it in spite of the Grand Canyon that stretched between us.

Upstairs my host is softly snoring, so I take the opportunity to indulge in a long, soaking bath and a shampoo. Who knows when I'll get the chance again?

Then I curl up on the sofa under the blanket Norman provided. Sleep will come hard, I know, so I don't fight for it, just let my mind wander loose. With so much going on what bubbles up to the surface comes as a surprise.

My cell phone.

It occurs to me that the call to deactivate it must have been made by a woman. Maybe Nina, although I can think of at least one other candidate.

Megan DeMarquess.

Chapter 8

MY FIRST day at AIA David had gone crazy and looped the sleeves of a boating sweater across his chest. Intercepting me in the aisle, he announced, "Found a case for you," with a mischievous smile.

"Wouldn't you just know," I pretended to complain. "You take a job, and right away they expect you to do some work."

David's lips squeezed together as he waved me into his office. We settled into our respective chairs before he spoke again. "Should be an easy start for you. A cervical strain and sprain."

"Once again, in English?"

The SIU manager's cheeks brightened to the red of that painting *Little Boy Blue*. "You have a lovely sense of humor," he remarked. "That should help with getting the insureds to open up."

"That or my terrible temper."

David's head reared back. "Oh no, no, no. Don't tell me that."

The subsequent silence warned me to shed the verbal body armor and plug into the moment.

"I wouldn't mind hearing more about getting our customers to open up."

David sighed, relief I suppose, before pondering the glass wall behind my head. "In a sense they're paying you to catch them in a lie," he explained. "To incriminate themselves, if you will. And if you're successful, they won't get any money out of us. Or anyway not as much as they want."

He studied the doorjamb for a moment before sharing his next thought. "Of course, compromise is sometimes more economical than going to court."

"Okay," I said, trying to learn. "Now what's this about a cervical strain and sprain?"

"Whiplash," he clarified. "A rear-ender Claims wants us to check out. Driver and victim both with AIA, and unfortunately the vic has full tort. He's after a ridiculous amount for pain and suffering—thirty thousand. You look as if you have a question."

More like a hundred and one, but what I asked was how he wanted me to proceed.

"Computer research first, interviews second. Keep the insured in mind, of course, but try not to do anything that will come back and bite us in the ass."

Megan DeMarquess's workplace was half a mile down a familiar back road I'd patrolled back on the job, at the time an overgrown lovers' lane for high school kids. Now it was two acres of truck-flattened dirt with a low brick building that had already lived a rough life. I shut the Taurus's windows tight against the dust and went inside.

The whole interior was office space, but the decor reminded me of a neighborhood bar—two vintage-style girlie calendars newly turned to November, a rusty street sign that said, "Lois Lane," a poster I recognized as last year's Villanova basketball schedule featuring a sweaty young stud dunking the ball. At my side were three wooden visitors' chairs and, front and center, a metal desk manned by a young female wearing a lightweight telephone headset. Behind her were four more desks, two with computers, three with middle-aged men all eying me as if I were a flying saucer but trying to be cool about it.

I approached the young woman. "I'm Lauren Beck from the Amalgamated Insurance Association. Might I have a word with you regarding your recent claim?"

The insured, Megan DeMarquess—who else could she be?—ripped off the headset and plumped up her medium brown mane with her free hand. So far she was pleased to see me, and I hoped to keep it that way.

"Mike," she addressed the youngest of the three men. "Coffee-break. Okay? I gotta talk to this woman here." He accepted the headset without taking his eyes off me.

Megan gestured toward the foul-smelling brew burbling in a pot on the back table. "Want some?"

"No thanks. You go ahead."

"Nah. Hasn't been agreeing with me. Wanna step outside to talk?"

We exited past the rest rooms and stood in the sun. The weather wasn't exactly wintery yet, but neither was it sunbathing warm.

I handed over my brand-new card to prove I was official. Then I asked for the basics, saving her social security number for last. With it I could check into her life even more extensively than I had this morning.

Megan asked a halfhearted, "Why?" and I replied that I was just making sure I had the right person.

She nodded her moony face to suggest that she'd got it, she was hip, she just thought she should ask, when in fact she probably should have refused. But hey, I wasn't her mother.

I jotted down the number while she lit a cigarette.

"Why don't you tell me what happened?" I began, sidestepping her exhaled smoke.

"I was waiting at a light, and my foot slipped," Megan told me. Then she took another drag and posed as if that was all she intended to say.

A dilemma. None of my previous employment experiences had required much in the way of finesse. It's true that in recent years police have been adopting a less adversarial, more public-friendly approach, but let's be honest here. A badge and a gun were usually all I'd needed to get answers out of people. Now, armed with nothing but a notebook, squared off against a twenty-two-year-old woman wearing KMart clothes and a hardened expression, I realized I needed to loosen up.

I stuck out my foot to relax my posture and mumbled, "These things happen, I guess." Then I remembered the tape recorder.

"Oh, shit," I blurted. "Mind if I record this? Sorry. It's my first case."

"Sure, go ahead." My ineptitude had melted her icy blue eyes just enough, so this time I relaxed for real.

"Here we go," I said, extending the blinking recorder in my hand. "I'm interviewing Megan DeMarquess on Tuesday, November fourth outside the Ajax Recycling Plant. Megan, can you please tell me how your car happened to hit the rear end of Mr. Tanner's car?"

She swung her hand to let the breeze take care of some cigarette ash. Then she started speaking in that self-conscious fashion you sometimes hear on your answering machine.

"My foot slipped," she said. "Is that okay?"

I told her yes, although I had no idea what the little recorder was capable of. "Did Mr. Tanner appear to be hurt when he got out of the car?"

"Oh, hell, no," she said, already forgetting about the recording. "Jimmy was mad, but I wouldn't say he looked hurt. I really don't think he should get any money for that."

"You call him Jimmy, so I take it you two are acquainted."

"No, not really."

"But you both used to live at 209 East Sixth Street in Landis..."

Megan raised the cigarette and extended her chin. "What's going on here? Why did you ask me that?"

Inappropriate anger, a trick liars love to death. I shrugged and tried to look ingenuous. "I'm just investigating the claim, that's all. It doesn't matter whether you knew him or not. I only figured you knew each other because you used to have the same address."

"Yeah, well, okay. We used to live together, and now we don't. Anyway that doesn't have anything to do with the accident. My foot slipped, that's all. Jimmy wasn't really hurt. Not bad anyway. I don't understand why you're asking me all these questions."

I did a little shrug/head tilt/pout combination. Then I said, "Money involved. Gotta put as much as I can in my report. So where were you going, if you don't mind my asking?"

"My sister's."

"And Jimmy just happened to be stopped at the light in front of you?"

"Yeah, really surprised the hell out of me. I guess that's why my foot slipped."

"Okay. Then what happened?"

Megan wrapped her long sweater tighter across her chest and stared over my shoulder while she reflected. "We got out of the cars. Me and Jimmy talked about it, then I left."

"Did the police come?"

"Yeah, Jimmy called them. They took down some stuff."

"Then you went to your sister's," I supplied. "Where's that?"

She rattled off the address of an apartment building in the Suncrest section of Landis. "You don't need to talk to her, do you?"

I performed another shrug. "Just getting whatever you've got." I said. "You hurt at all?"

"No."

"Get a quote on your car?"

"Yeah, it's getting fixed next week." She waved her cigarette toward the back of the employee parking lot. From my research I recognized the plate number on the back of a black, four-year-old Toyota.

"Okay. I'll do my best to finish this up real soon."

"That'd be nice," Megan remarked, then thought about it and added, "I guess."

She dropped her cigarette and put it out with the toe of her shoe. Then she disappeared into the building, leaving me to either follow or walk around to my car alone.

I chose the latter, grinning with satisfaction all the way.

Megan DeMarquess had lied to me by omission, and I knew it. Knew it with profound certainty. Knew it as well as I knew my own name. I hadn't been so sure about anything since before I got sick.

Which was why I decided to roll with the feeling and go spy on her ex-boyfriend, Jimmy Tanner, the whiplash victim himself.

Chapter 9

Not terribly far from the three-hundred-store mall in King of Prussia is the more modest Meadow Woods Shopping Center. Also adjacent to Route 202, it offers an eclectic group of twenty varied enterprises intent on serving the surrounding office buildings during lunch hour, happy hour, and the even happier holiday shopping season.

James "Jimmy" Tanner worked at the Denmark Deli at the north end of the row. My uphill parking space offered a view of both the front and rear exits, but especially of the long glass wall along the side.

For a guy wearing a foam-rubber collar, Jimmy moved pretty quickly, but it was approaching noon and business was brisk. After twenty minutes, I decided I was hungry, too, and that maybe it was time for me to make the victim's acquaintance.

"Turkey, Swiss, lettuce, tomato, and honey mustard on whole wheat," I told him when my turn came. There was a tray slide made of steel tubing and fruit salads and juices on ice as you went along. I chose Rosenberger's chocolate milk and an apple while I was waiting.

Young Jim stood perhaps six-feet tall. His skin was pasty and marred by a few blemishes. His eyes were protuberant green edged with pale brown to match his hair. He wore a dark brown collared golf shirt with the deli's name discreetly stitched in yellow, and when you factored in the cervical collar, he looked as if he were aspiring to become a giraffe.

"What happened to your neck?" I inquired.

"Car accident," he replied, sizing me up as if he might need to recognize me later.

"Hurt much?"

"Comes and goes. You got some interest in me, or are you just being nosy?"

"A little of both. I'm with Amalgamated..."

Jimmy handed me my wrapped sandwich, didn't even ask if it was for here or to go. "Talk to my lawyer," he said with finality. "Next!"

One more thing David might have thought to mention—that the victim might be represented.

"Fine," I said as if things were completely copasetic. "Who's your lawyer?"

Jimmy glanced up from the provolone he was placing over some salami and recited the name of a TV ambulance chaser.

I paid the cashier then returned to the driver's seat of the Taurus to eat. Too much mustard and the chocolate milk could have been chillier, but most of my attention was on Jimmy anyway. I had my company-issued Minolta all set for motion and was waiting to see if he stepped outside for a break after the lunch rush subsided. Maybe I would get a shot of him carrying something heavy.

One thirty was soon ticking toward two, and I was bored. I began to bet with myself whether the people getting out of their cars were headed for Eberly Electronics just beyond the deli or if they were merely late for lunch.

It was a lousy game; so when a truck backed up to the electronics' store's back door and two men began to load it, I switched. Televisions, stereo equipment, DVD players, washers, dryers—I tried to guess the contents of each box, then checked myself by reading the labels through the zoom lens of the camera.

Finally, finally I caught a break. I had the Minolta in place and was scoping out a DVD box when Jimmy emerged from the deli carrying two green trash bags. I was so excited that I almost forgot to turn on the camera, but I managed to get a perfect thirty seconds of the whiplash victim lugging the trash across the rear driveway, lifting the bags, and throwing them into the dumpster.

A knock on my window startled a yelp out of me followed by a four-letter word.

"Hey you!" a menacing voice shouted. "Get the fuck outta here." One of the men who'd been loading the truck, the one who could lift washing machines all by himself. This close he looked very large and very angry.

I considered trying to explain myself, but the guy was yelling "goddamn spying bitch" and pulling at my door handle. When it wouldn't open, he began to kick the car.

"Okay, okay," I shouted. I threw the camera onto the passenger seat and reached for the ignition key.

"Don't come back," the electronics thug threatened as he punched my window again.

"Leaving now," I warned in case the guy needed to move his foot.

My last glimpse was of Jimmy Tanner giving the thug one of those "Thanks, man, I owe you one" nods.

Chapter 10

I awake to the smell of toast.

The sofa I'm on is scratchy, and I recall with a jolt that I've imposed on Dad's dear friend, Norman.

Glad that I had the foresight to sleep in a sweat suit, I throw off the covers and ease myself upright.

"Morning," I call toward the kitchen before I trot upstairs.

My host grunts and utters something that sounds hung-over. When I finally join him, his normally cherubic face looks almost sinister.

"Toast okay?" From his seat at the table he waves a buttered slice in the air. "Usually I have toast."

"Toast is fine, but I'll cook something else if you want. That is, if you have anything around."

"Eggs? Haven't had eggs in a while."

"You got it." The expiration date on the carton is only a couple days past, so I take out a frying pan and start melting butter.

On the table beside the man who is perhaps my Dad's best friend sits another tumbler of Long Island iced tea, which brings into question a couple of formerly insignificant details. Norman is perpetually late. Norman will not schedule anything before ten a.m., and then he will be late. Norman prefers to let someone else drive because he has a remarkably bad history with automobiles.

Okay, so dear old Uncle Norman is alcoholic. My childhood memories of him are suddenly at risk, until I remind myself they are *childhood* memories. Both of us have been adults for some time now.

He waves the tumbler in my direction. "You want a little hair of the dog to go with?"

"No thanks, Norm," I answer gently. "Gotta be sharp for work."

He avoids my eyes as he lifts the tumbler to his lips, but it's impossible to miss the regret he's attempting to hide. One glance would show him that it's my regret, too– my sweet, funny, honorary uncle has suddenly become an ordinary man with flaws like everybody else.

But that's not all. Just by being here, I've diminished him.

Which is why, as soon as I place two perfect, over-light eggs in front of him and sit down behind mine, I ask if I might tell him about my problems.

Norman's chin jerks and his eyes blink, and in that split second I read surprise laced with joy, validation, gratitude.

"Sure, Jellybean," he says. "I'm all ears." He flicks one of the jug-handles on the side of his head to make me laugh; and when I do, his smile stretches wider.

After I finish my list of woes, Norman sets down his fork and wipes his lips with a napkin.

Then he tilts his stubbly chin. "Think it was something you said?"

I just about choke before I can respond. "Maybe. Jeez, I didn't think of that. Maybe."

Norman's face has gone pink. "I was just joshing you, kid. You know that, right? Don't take me serious."

"I know, I know. But all kidding aside. You might be onto something."

"You lost me. What're we talking about?"

"The day Nina threw Corinne's CEA report at me."

His raised eyebrows said, "And...?"

"And I completely freaked out."

YES OR *no*. That's what I'd been contemplating all the way home from my final job interviews at AIA. *Yes*, work for more money doing the investigative work I love, or *No thanks*, I've got other priorities right now. Corinne was totally onboard with the former, but what she recommended didn't make sense.

When I let myself into the kitchen, Nina was lifting a tray loaded with tea and fruitcake for Corinne's afternoon snack.

"Want me to take that up?" I offered.

"Why?"

"Don't you have to get home to Jilly?"

"Yeh, at *three forty-five*," as if I was supposed to know her kid's school-bus schedule.

"Okay, that's cool," I conceded. "You and your mother don't get that much time together."

Nina set down the tray. "I will now." She had adopted the stance of a spectator, the same amused expression, too.

"What do you mean?"

"Jilly and I are moving in."

The floor shifted under my feet. My heart raced. My skin beaded with sweat. Somehow, don't ask me how, I took a breath and arranged my face into a semblance of happy surprise.

"Good," I lied. "That's good."

"Somebody needs to look after my mother."

My silence said it all.

"You didn't think you...You did, didn't you?" Nina actually laughed out loud, not a sound I was eager to hear again soon. "Admit it. That's what you thought."

Furious would have been one way to play it, but I managed to keep control. "Yes, that's what I thought," I told her, "and why shouldn't I? It's my chance to repay her for what she did for me."

"Because you two are so close."

"Well, yes. She's almost been like my..." Face flaming, I waited for it.

"... mother?"

Eviscerating me wasn't enough. Nina walked over to her purse and reached in. Extracted a folded paper. Dangled it in front of me.

"You feel like a daughter to her? Here. Deal with this."

It was Corinne's latest CEA test results, the carcinoembryonic antigen blood test that tells your doctor who's winning—you or the cancer. The figure on the page took my breath away.

Corinne's treatments were not working.

My back stiffened and my fists clenched. I wanted to scream or cry or break something.

Nina watched with tormented eyes of her own, but there was a difference. Her emotions were permitted; mine were not. Corinne had been clear about that, and like an aftershock I finally understood why.

I knew too much. To her, my face would be as damning as the figures on the printout and just as difficult to live with. Either I had to bury my new knowledge deep–immediately–or learn how to fake it fast.

I dropped the printout and stumbled out the door.

The lobby of Soames Memorial Hospital was the same desperately upbeat peach and green it had been when I was a patient; only the pumpkin flower arrangement on the Information desk was new. I had paused to catch my breath just inside the entrance, and the elderly volunteer met my eyes with an eager smile. I waved her off with a body-language, "Thanks, but I know where I'm going."

And I did, only too well--Chemotherapy Suite, second floor, third door on the right. Evidently, the snack machine wasn't working again, because a man in a green sweater and jeans was banging it with the heel of his hand, projecting all his pent-up anguish into the failed purchase of some peanut-butter crackers. When a passing candy-striper touched his arm and whispered into his ear, he blushed and glanced around and hurried to take a seat.

I knew this because I had circumvented the small registration desk to stand in the aisle between two short rows of chairs. I didn't dare insinuate myself into the treatment room, so that was as far as I could go.

I was trying to decide whether to sign in and take a seat when a familiar nurse stepped into view. She finished ushering an elderly man back to a chair, and before she could hurry away I called her name.

"Amy." In the silence, it sounded like a shout. "I'm Lauren Beck," I reminded her. "Do you have a moment to talk about Corinne Wilder?"

The nurse was about my height, five seven, and had gorgeous aqua-blue eyes. Stunning eyes. Also black hair curlier than mine but not as long.

Amy smiled with recognition. "I didn't realize you're related to Corinne. How are you?"

"Terrific," I answered, letting the relationship error go. "Just worried about her."

"If she's having problems, she should get in touch with her doctor. Maybe come back in." Standard advice the oncology nurse recited every day of the week.

"No!"

The nurse's head jerked. Magazines lowered. Faces swiveled to stare. My chest was heaving. I was losing my grip.

I wiped a tear. "No. It isn't that."

Amy steered me into the hall, but hospitals offer about as much privacy as an ant farm. Not five feet from us a woman was futzing around inside the open window of the pharmacy.

Screw it. "Corinne isn't getting better," I blurted. "Something is seriously wrong."

"What makes you say that?"

The answer was personal experience. By the third round of chemo I was sick sick sick. And weak. And nearly bald. I couldn't eat because the interior of my mouth was sore, and so was my stomach. *All* fast-growing cells are attacked by the drugs. You about die before you're brought back to life.

But an oncology nurse knew all that, so I told her that Corinne *wasn't* very ill, that she ate normally, and that she hadn't lost any hair that I could see.

"Different people react differently to the chemo." Another stock answer.

"No," I argued. "No! Don't you see? The dosage must be wrong or something. *Nothing is happening.*"

Amy, patted the air and lowered her voice. "Hold on now, Ms. Beck. Think about what you're saying."

"Think about it! Think about it?"

She was right, of course. My frustration was speaking instead of my head.

The nurse huffed out a sigh. "What's the matter with you today?" she challenged. "Where's that fantastic attitude you had when it was happening to you? You fought like hell—remember?"

"Corinne taught me...She was the reason..." Clenching my teeth, I fished a tissue out of my purse. Wiped the mascara from under my eyes. Blew my nose.

"So now she needs you to have that attitude for her."

I locked onto the other woman's amazing blue eyes and tried my best to sound convincing. "She can't be getting better," I insisted. "Don't you see? She isn't getting worse, so how can she be getting better?"

A rustling sound reminded us that we weren't entirely alone. The pharmacist was eavesdropping her ass off.

Amy shooed me further down the hall.

"Go to her, Lauren," she advised. "Pull yourself together and go see her. You'll feel better and so will she."

"I don't get it," Norman confesses. He has replenished his tumbler with ice cubes and booze, yet he's sober enough that I don't dismiss his confusion. "You think the nurse is mad at you?"

"No."

"Who then?"

Deflated, I admit, "I guess I don't know. Somebody who heard my accusations? Somebody they told?"'

Norman makes a waffling motion with his head. "What else you got, kid?"

So I switch to describing my suspicions about Bob Battersby, then Megan DeMarquess, her ex-boyfriend and his thugs. Yet the back of my mind reverberates with the emotion I vented in the hospital hallway. Multiple pebbles were thrown into the pond that day, and the rings continued to overlap and spread.

After I left the hospital, I had climbed into my own personal cocoon, my red Miata. The paint was dull and full of dings, plus there was a rust patch near the right rear tire. Back when I was a working cop, I'd bought the used convertible for therapy—carefree, windblown release, precisely what I needed to deal with Corinne's terrifying CEA count.

For over an hour I pacified my mind with the streets of Landis, the small city I know so well. Only when the late-autumn sun sliced sideways through the brilliant poplars and ash and oak did I finally head home. When I pulled into Corinne's short driveway, the kitchen light was already on.

The house itself is nothing special, just pale green aluminum siding with white trim. Inside the living-room, dining area and kitchen are all in one with a peninsula of appliances to divide the work space from the rest. Shelves on the far wall were filled cheek to jowl with those bizarre cookie jars staring across at a collection of sports-figure bobble-heads gleaned from various fast-food promotions. I'd lived there four years and still wasn't sure if I was supposed to admire the eyesores or laugh at them.

Corinne rested under a comforter on the living room sofa.

"Hey," I greeted her.

"Umph," she replied, sitting up and turning my way.

When I told Amy, the nurse, that the chemotherapy hadn't affected Corinne, I'd exaggerated. She had lost flesh and energy, the sparkle in her eye, the stamina to snap back at me. I sorely missed seeing her cheeks pink up when she laughed, missed watching those graceful hands caress a favorite possession.

"Put another CD on, will you?" she requested, and I hastened to comply.

"What's your pleasure? Volero? Conway Twitty? Hip Hop?"

"Loon Summer, I think. It feels like winter already."

I located her selection and placed it in the still-warm tray. Then I returned Beethoven to the rack while an almost tuneless New Age fluty thing began to summon visions of ducks on a lake and water sloshing against the side of a canoe.

I took a chair across from my housemate.

"So where'd you go?" she inquired.

"Went to visit a friend," I fibbed.

"Oh, really?" Corinne's amusement was tainted with irony. "A sick friend?"

We stared at each other for an awkward moment. Then Corinne said, "You had a fight with Nina, didn't you? That's why you ran off."

"No. No!" I protested. Technically, Nina and I hadn't disagreed at all. Yet the fact that Corinne had detected tension between us was just below her CEA count when it came to bad news.

"I was driving around. Clearing my head. That's all." This, at least, was something I'd done before, something Corinne could allow herself to believe.

"She told you she's moving in, didn't she?"

"Yes."

"You going to be okay with that?"

"Of course. I think it's a great idea."

Corinne sighed with relief. "She's between jobs, you know."

So that was how we were playing it, the post-divorce, money-is-tight card. Fine.

Even still, I felt a small chill, just the touch of a snowflake. Corinne and I had stopped being completely honest with each other.

Chapter 11

I left Norman alone with his Long Island iced tea, but I shouldn't have come to work. I'm still numb, functioning purely by rote. But where else do I have to go?

"What's wrong?" David's voice startles me as I boot up my computer.

I tell him about Corinne without tears, but just barely.

"You want to take some time?" Today's pastel green shirt makes him look almost as bad as I feel. But maybe I'm projecting.

"No, I think I'll soldier on." Corinne wanted my dad to be pragmatic about her death; and if he could manage it, I should at least try.

"Your call," David tells me.

He turns to leave, but I forestall him. "There's something I've been meaning to ask."

"Oh?" David seems pleased, almost flattered.

"Do the insureds ever try to retaliate?"

My manager scratches his blonde head. "Like how?"

"Like maybe following you the way you followed them?"

"Did something like that happen?"

"Friday night." I describe my encounter with the pickup truck.

David rubs his cheek with his knuckles while he gives that some thought. His conclusion: "Sounds more like a weekend thing to me." End of subject.

He gestures toward the computer. "If you're sure you want to stay, check out the case I just gave you. Possible arson. Got a specialist taking care of the technical stuff, but I thought you might like to do the interviews."

Motive. Opportunity. For once I know what he's talking about.

The assignment does look interesting—a travel agency in a former residence—so I begin to poke around online. Soon I have confirmation that Jerry Shumacher's Getaway Vacations has indeed been circling the drain for three quarters in a row. Even Pollyanna would have flagged the fire insurance claim for closer inspection.

I'm printing out the particulars in my carpeted cubbyhole when I get a call originating from Ajax Recycling Plant, the place where Megan DeMarquess works.

"Ms. Beck?"

"Hey, Megan," I reply. "What can I do for you?"

"I've been thinking about Jimmy's claim, you know, that I hit him and all. And I think maybe he's right. You should pay him whatever he wants."

Part of me is thinking *Isn't that sweet—they're back together,* while my rational side says, *No way, Jose.*

"Well, Megan," I stall. "I'll certainly consider your opinion, but I just gather the facts," and I don't have all of them yet, "Somebody else decides whether AIA will pay or not."

"Oh, okay. Maybe I should talk to them."

"I'm sorry. Your claims adjuster makes that determination, but he's not in the office right now." Not in this office anyway. "Then the lawyers might become involved."

We hang up, neither of us satisfied.

I shut off the computer and retrieve my purse from the drawer. Right now I might not have enough focus to interview everybody within sight of a suspected arson scene today, but at least I can talk to Megan's sister.

My destination, Suncrest, is a poorly planned section of Landis maintained in the crumbling style of Rome. It has sidewalks, but no yards, and parking is done on the diagonal. Tracy Lune's building, a tall white block of cement, tucks up against a commercial bakery, which bellies up to a dry cleaning plant, which towers over a row of ancient duplexes.

The battery of mailboxes confirms that Megan's older sibling lives on the first floor in unit #2, but the label gives no hint of a husband.

"Come in," a blousy blonde responds to my knock while the toddler on her hip eyes me suspiciously. Nearby stands a bright-eyed four-year-old boy.

"You're really here about that little fender bender?" Megan's sister inquires.

I remind her that an injury occurred. I do not mention the disproportionately large lawsuit.

"Oh, that." She usheres me into a long rectangular living room smelling of cigarette ash and soiled diaper. A sofa and chair set in blue and white is surrounded by an assortment of toys. White drapes overhang the floor, and posters of rural New England are tastefully arranged on the walls. Ms. Lune might be broke and divorced, but she's holding it all together.

"Coffee?" she offers.

"How about if we just sit for a few minutes and get this over with...unless you'd like to change that diaper first."

Narrowed eyes. "Not if this'll only take a minute."

"Right," I reply, and we all sit down.

"I like your car," the boy announces.

I smile my appreciation of the comment but address his mother. "Can you please tell me what you know about Megan's evening before she arrived here?"

Tracy lifts a hand. "They had dinner."

"Hold on a second." Once again, I forgot the tape recorder, so I dig it out, rattle off the who, what, and where, then put it on the coffee table between us. "Go ahead."

Mom is about to speak, but her son beats her to it. "Where'd you get those shoes?" I've got on Bass saddle-style dirty bucks and brown argyles.

"A, um, shoe store." The child seems to expect more, so I add, "Thank you for asking."

"Megan asked for our mother's pot roast recipe," Tracy continues. "She thought they were getting back together."

"Oh? How'd that go?"

"You have holes in your ears but you don't have any earrings."

"Joey, do Mommy a favor and shut up for a couple minutes, okay? Not very well," Tracy answers. "Megan was all set for a romantic evening, you know? But nine o'clock Jimmy pushes back from the table and says he's gotta go. Megan thought he meant like to the john or something, but he meant *go*, as in leave."

"Not good," I observe.

"Not good at all," Tracy agrees.

"So was Megan furious, or what?"

"I have a loose tooth. See?"

"Joey!...Not exactly furious. More like disappointed."

I'm not buying it. "Upset?"

"No. Megan isn't like that. She was hurt, that's all."

"Okay. Then what?"

"Well, you know. She was driving over here and Jimmy's car was stopped at a light and she was so surprised she ran right into him."

The latter sounds awfully familiar, but of course Megan and Tracy are sisters, and sisters talk to each other. Some of them at least.

"What was Megan like when she got here?"

"*Then* she was upset."

"Scared upset? Sorry upset? Worried about what the accident would cost upset?"

"Yeah. She was pretty much a mess."

"Rrrrrrr." Joey runs his miniature front-loader across my dirty buck, but it's only a low-grade blip on my consciousness screen. I'm consumed by an insight that feels so right it almost has to be true.

I show Tracy what I hope passes for knowing concern. "I had a fender-bender like Megan's once. Nothing much happened to my car, but it really shook me up. I ached all over for days. Hated driving for a while. You think that's what it's been like for your sister?"

"Yeah," Tracy concurs, "probably."

"Lucky she didn't lose the baby," I remark, as if I actually know something.

The toddler presently asleep on Tracy's hip rises and falls with her mother's shrug. "If you call that luck."

Chapter 12

I feel no better for guessing correctly that Megan DeMarques is pregnant; that's her own joy or despair and none of mine. But I do return to the office annoyed by her dishonesty. Not that it materially changes the nature of her claim or Jimmy's. Suspicious as their behaviors are, I doubt that I can deny them with what I've got so far.

After I sign onto my computer, I glance around the SIU unit to check what's going on. David is absent, the coffee pot cold. Only Bob Battersby and a giant man clad in catalog chinos and an electric blue shirt stand in the aisle apparently talking business.

Battersby must have felt my eyes on him, though, because now he's looking my way. His cold expression is a deliberate snub, so I counter with the kind of smile I know he'll hate as much as much as I hate his chauvinism—if that is all it is.

In and around Glendenning county the name Beck sometimes stirs up resentment. Could be my dad sold someone's family farm, or my brother beat out the wrong nephew in lacrosse. Maybe I arrested somebody's boyfriend or their adored Uncle Sid. Throw in the male egos I've been told I crushed—by accident or design—and I probably should run around town in a flak jacket.

I don't know what's bugging Bob Battersby, but it's high time for me to find out. Somehow.

After the computer and I get caught up on the approaching weather—wind and rain—and my horoscope, which advises me to "keep to myself," I walk around to contemplate the coffee urn.

A burly body suddenly looms over me, the six-foot-five, blue-shirted giant. His eyes are also blue, bedded in endearing pillows of flesh, hair an even mix of black and white.

"Mike Thomas," he says, offering me a bear paw. "Car theft."

I introduce myself as "Whatisname's replacement," then state my name.

"An improvement," the large man concludes. "Big improvement."

"How can you tell?"

"Trained observer. Know how to operate this thing?" He gestures toward David's intimidating coffeemaker.

"Nope. You?" Cute, likeable guy. Also married.

He rummages around in a cabinet and scores a large white coffee filter, which in his hand looks like a bon-bon cup. From the refrigerator he extracts a pound bag of the expensive grind-it-yourself stuff David favors and begins to scoop. While he counts, his mouth takes little guppy breaths.

Sensing my gaze, he pauses long enough to hand me the machine's carafe. "You mind filling that?" He gestures toward the water cooler.

When the deed is done, he motions me into a chair near his own oversized accommodation, puts his feet up, and asks me how things are going. I notice that his chin has a nick from this morning's shave, and he's unconsciously tapping his wedding ring against his head.

I tell him I feel as if I've been thrown into the deep end of the pool.

"Can you swim?"

"I used to be a cop."

"Well, then, no problemo. Whatcha working on?"

I mention my whiplash case. "Ever deal with that TV lawyer, Alex Kensington?"

"Who hasn't?" the auto-theft specialist muses.

"Me."

"Oh, right."

"So what can I expect?"

Coffee fumes are wafting our way, and Mike draws in a sizeable sniff. "Personal injury cases usually settle for three times the medical costs, okay?" he says with his exhale.

"Okay."

"So you can expect him to send his boy to every specialist in the book—x-rays, MRI, therapy out the wazoo. Anything to raise the ante."

"Is that normal?"

"For that scumbag it is."

"Anything I can do about it?"

"Prove the vic isn't hurt, or anyway not *very* hurt."

I tell him I got that yesterday. "Carrying trash bags."

Mike waves his oversized head. "Kensington'll just claim the kid had a good day.

"What else can I tell you?"

I glance around, but my nemesis is nowhere in sight. "This isn't related to a case, but I need to know whether Bob Battersby hates women in general or just me."

"Seriously?"

"Yes, seriously. Do you think you can find out? Discreetly?"

Mike blinks while he gauges the degree of unpleasantness. "We don't really socialize."

I nod without apology. "Some scary shit's been happening to me."

"You think…?"

I shrug.

His mind made up, Mike spreads his hands in a priestly fashion. "Consider it done."

A phone begins to ring. "That's me," the car-theft investigator says, and he's gone.

So now, thanks to my new friend, Mike, I know I need more proof that Jimmy Tanner can do things he shouldn't be able to do. I also have an idea of how to get it.

After fortifying myself with "homemade" vegetable beef soup and a floury biscuit down at the basement food court--I venture out into the weather, which, as predicted, is no longer nice. All of eastern Pennsylvania, all that I can see, has become a dreary watercolor--pigeon-gray mist, wind ripping the last autumn leaves from the maples, rattling whatever brown curls still cling to the oaks. Not a day to sit in your car watching somebody make sandwiches through a window.

A glance into the Denmark Deli as I drive by reveals that Tanner is still wearing his cervical collar, also that there isn't much of a demand for sandwiches this afternoon.

Intending to circle around the rear of the mall to the front customer lot, I turn left at the dumpster; but the electronic store's delivery van blocks my way. Wearing only shirtsleeves, the thug from yesterday is busy wheeling a refrigerator up a loading ramp.

"Hey!" he shouts.

I brake, back up, then shift into forward as the driver jumps out and takes a few threatening strides toward me. I steer around him and escape along the back of the stores, but I'm thinking *Why?* Why get all grouchy over a whiplash claim filed by a kid who works next door? One more question without an answer.

Around front I park near the jewelry store--facing the lot's exit just in case--and climb out to have a look around.

Jimmy's dented blue Neon sits beside a brown SUV in the employees' row, the one least convenient to the stores.

Now what? Nearly two-thirty, the deli's closing time, dozens of cars, but no people in sight. Why not?

The gusting wind numbs my hands and ears, but the grassy edge of the blacktop offers just what I need--a generous selection of shale. My dad tried to winnow the stuff out of his fields over time but still hit rock every time he sank a shovel. Finding a small pointy piece to let the air out of Jimmy's tire takes about thirty seconds.

I choose Jimmy's right front wheel because the SUV on the driver's side leaves me an impossible camera shot. Squatted down, I keep an eye on my surroundings. Motorists on the highway can see me, but at sixty miles an hour what can they do?

The chore seems to take forever, and by the time the tire's flat my fingers are so frozen I can scarcely screw the cap back on the nozzle. Just standing up and relieving my cramped knees is a joy.

Oops. Two rows over a woman is getting into a white sedan. I hold my breath and keep watch and thank heaven that she pulls out without ever glancing my way.

Then I run to retrieve the camera, quickly hide behind a green van the size of a garden shed. No question, I would love to watch for Jimmy in the warmth and safety of my car, but I don't dare. On foot if something threatens to ruin my photo op, I can easily adjust. In the car I'll be stuck, and there will be no repeat performance.

So I wait. Anytime I see movement, I pretend the van is mine and fuss inside my purse. Mostly I hover around the rear door toward the highway with the camera around my neck, only ducking out of the wind when I begin to shiver.

Jimmy emerges about half-past three. Rubbing his hands together and humming nothing anybody would recognize, he stops dead when he sees the tire.

The boy certainly knows how to curse. From my vantage point I prepare to photograph him opening his trunk, extracting equipment, tugging the lug nuts loose, pumping up the jack, removing the tire...all that wonderful stuff.

Except that isn't what he does. Still cursing, slapping his thighs with vexation, he turns on his heel and marches his ass into Eberly Electronics. A moment later out comes the electronics thug shrugging into a light jacket. He follows Jimmy back to the Neon, whereupon *he* lifts the trunk, extracts the lug wrench and the base of the jack, and *he* begins to address the problem—all while Jimmy stands by with his arms folded, neck all snug and warm inside his cervical collar.

The electronics thug has just asked Jimmy to hold the wrench when a voice behind me shouts, "Is this the broad you was talking about?"

I'm in motion before I exhale; but the delivery-truck driver--or whoever the squealer is--gets his fingers on my sleeve. I karate chop his hand and run.

Electronics Thug cuts the angle between me and the Taurus. Scarcely two yards from safety, his arms surround my shoulders. Breath smelling of German bologna hisses into my ear. "I told you..." His left hand grabs something he knows will hurt.

"Uncle Bill, let her go," Jimmy Tanner orders, dropping the lug wrench to the ground.

"Yeah, but..." Electronics Thug—Bill—doesn't want to release me. I consider stomping his foot and elbowing his stomach; but there is an interesting confidence in

Jimmy's oncoming stride, and I want to see how it plays out.

"I'll take it from here," the kid tells his uncle when he gets close. Forget about the blemished, puppy face, his expression is as hard as Bill's biceps.

"You sure, because I could...?"

"I'm sure."

"You're making a mistake," the older man warns, his abrupt release almost throwing me down.

Jimmy dips his head and stands pat until finally, finally, the older man stalks off.

The kid begins to crowd me backwards. "I don't know what you think you're doing," he says so close I can feel the heat of his skin, "but you're gonna stay away from me, you understand? I got a lawyer, and I got them." He refers to his uncle and the side of beef helping him work the jack, both of whom for some reason bow to his wishes. "So *leave me the fuck alone*. You hear?"

I slouch back to my car as if I'm chastened and chagrined, because I feel chastened and chagrined.

Never mind that Jimmy's bravado makes him appear every bit as dishonest as his ex-girlfriend–I still can't prove that either one of them is committing fraud.

Which harkens back to Cop School 101: Start at the scene of the crime.

Why not? It isn't as if I have somewhere better to go.

Chapter 13

Since Landis's Main Street is so familiar, I usually just veg out waiting for the lights to turn. Today I actually notice the brick sidewalk and the ginkgo trees, the bin of used books outside The Book Worm, the Spaulding basketballs displayed next to the aqua and green uniform trunks of my alma mater, Landis High. Across from Whorley's sporting goods the office supply store is now a Baby Gap, and our grand old Woolworth building seems to be empty again.

I parallel park four slots before the corner of Main and Duluth, feed the meter a quarter, and walk ahead to Bernie's Bistro. It will have been open at nine-thirty the night the accident occurred, so anyone looking out the window at the right moment would have seen everything.

From the corner vestibule, I take in the small round tables, dark wood, and ornate brass. No ferns, just lots of framed, oversized Toulouse Lautrec knock-offs. The type of food is anybody's guess, but you can bet it will be trendy.

"'ello, 'ello." The proprietor, Bernard Romaine, waves me inside. His black hair is slicked back from a widow's peak, serving to accentuate his nose. Dressed in a gray shirt and pants with gleaming accessories, he exudes authority; but wearing anything else he could be mistaken for a flabby tourist, an impression he has taken pains to avoid.

I tell him my name and why I'm here. "Did you happen to see the accident that took place out front on the evening of October 24?"

"Ack," the bistro's owner snorts. "You sound like TV. Everybody love Bernie. Talk like you love Bernie, too. Comma in and have a beer."

"Okay, why not?"

He guides me to the table closest to the cash register and offers me an end chair, keeping a view of the whole room for himself.

"Carlo, Sam Adams draft, please," he tells a waiter wrapped in a white apron. "Two."

As soon as we're served, the proprietor leans forward in a friendly fashion. "So what you need from Bernie?" he inquires.

I set my mini-recorder on the table between us, and he gestures toward it by way of permission. "Did you see the accident I mentioned?"

"I did. I did," my host answers with a nod, and my pulse picks up.

"You did? You personally?"

"Oh, yes. A most amusing event."

"Where exactly were you standing, if I may ask?"

The bistro owner jabs at the air behind him with his left elbow. "Minding the money and the door, same as always."

The cashier's booth is slightly raised, so he would have had an excellent view of Megan and Jimmy's little fender-bender through the wall-to-wall front window.

"What about the door?" I worry. Solid oak and centered in the corner, it obscured the traffic light.

"A pleasant evening," Bernie replies with a twinkle in his eye. "It was open for to seduce the customer."

Convinced that he has everything I need, I return his mischievous smile. Still, it appears that prying the candy out of Poppa's hand will require both guile and patience, so I sip my beer while I plan my own seduction.

"The young man," I begin. "His car was first in line waiting for the light?"

Bernie makes a pfh sound and gestures with his fingers. "A boy merely. He had no..." he rubs his chin and consults the ceiling. I figure he wants to say cojones or some other foreign word equally as off-color.

I assure him that I get it. "But his Dodge Neon was first in line, right?"

A nod.

"And the young woman drove up behind him at what speed would you say?"

"No speed."

"No speed? I'm sorry. What do you mean?"

The proprietor swivels his tush around and points to a spot a few car lengths down the block. "She stopped back dare."

Tight with anticipation, he waits, waits...and finally I catch on.

We share a grin; but I need him to say it aloud, so I tilt my head to indicate the tape recorder.

"Awright, awright. She stopped back dare, then vroom, vroom, boom—she hitsa his car." For emphasis, he punches the table and splashes some beer.

"Then what?"

Reaching for a napkin, my host waves his head. "Dey fight," he says, "ona sidewalk." He points to a spot ten feet to the left of the bistro's door.

"Any pushing or shoving?"

"Yelling is all. 'You so and so,' things like that."

"You remember any specific words?"

"You don' wanna hear."

I nod toward the recorder again. "Yes, actually, I do."

Reluctantly, Bernie complies. "'You crazy, goddamn bitch,'" he quotes. "'Why you fuckin' go an do dat?'"

"That's all?"

"Yeah, yeah. All I hear."

I shut off the tape, then I tell him, "You're right, Bernie—I do love you."

He grins as if he's been waiting all day to hear that. "Howa you like you steak?" he asks. "'Ona me," he adds.

The offer is more welcome than he could ever know, and once again the man is right. His marinated skirt steak and parmesan fries turn out to be the best meal I've had in ages.

Mellowed by beer and warm food, I tip the server and thank the bistro owner profusely. Then it's out into the chilly black night for me.

Then I remember, and a white-hot fury consumes me. Standing stock-still on the sidewalk, I let it roil.

There is nowhere for me to go. Maybe if Corinne were still here, or my dad...but no.

So be it.

I return to the Taurus, open the door, put the key in the ignition.

Why waste a perfectly good rage? Why not dump some of it on Megan DeMarquess?

Chapter 14

My notes told me Megan lives in Landis at 314 East Tulip Drive, Apartment B, a front corner of a stucco quad with rear parking. I leave the Taurus and make a quick circuit of the place on foot. No dented black Toyota in the alley. Mail bulging out of her box. No light coming from the unit labeled B.

Rather than wait in my frigid car, I decide to look for the insured elsewhere. Her attempt to get AIA to settle in her boyfriend's favor suggests that she might be with him.

A convenient two point three miles away, Jimmy's place—number 5545—falls in the middle of a block-long rectangle of attached brick homes. Some of the others have wrought-iron railings by their doorsteps, or flowerboxes, or plastic toys on the small square of lawn between the door and the sidewalk. Fifty-five forty-five is distinguished by nothing.

Here, you park on the street or you don't park. After two trips around the block, I finally snag a slot with a view of the accident victim's door. Jimmy's blue Neon sits only a few paces away; and as I suspected, Megan's Toyota is tucked around the corner questionably close to a fire hydrant.

Twiddling my thumbs in a freezing car until she emerges from Jimmy's bachelor pad would be foolish, especially since that might not happen until morning. Anyway, if they're working together, it doesn't matter if he hears what I have to say.

Jumping from foot to foot to get warm, I give his door a polite knock. And again, but all that gets me is barked knuckles. After a minute I figure the hell with it and hammer with my fist. I'm about to start kicking the door with my heel when suddenly it opens, surprising me so much I almost forget to switch on the mini-recorder concealed in my left hand. Never mind permission; this recording is insurance for me.

"Now what do you want?" Tanner demands. He has on socks, jeans, and a crewneck Flyers sweatshirt. Apparently cervical collars aren't something you wear to bed, because I'm seeing his throat for the first time.

I tell him I'm there to speak with Megan.

"We been through all this. She's not..."

"I'm here," she contradicts him from the edge of the room. "It's okay, Jimmy. I called her today."

"Mind if I step inside?" I ask. "It's cold out here."

I'm allowed to slip through the door, but that's where the hospitality ends.

"So they going to pay, or what?" Megan must have grabbed the first clothes that came to hand–slippers and a man's bathrobe. Her brown mane is fluffed to the max, and I'm annoyed to see that she hasn't quit smoking. Mommy dearest, in training.

"Or what, Megan," I state. "Mainly because you rammed into Jimmy's car on purpose."

Testosterone driven male that he is, Tanner lurches at me.

"Jimmy!" Megan shouts, but he shakes off her hand and crowds closer.

I resist giving up ground because I'm stubborn. I'd rather not be so near those long, ape-like arms, but I'm quick and I've been trained. Unless Jimmy-boy's a martial-art whiz, I'll probably be okay.

Behind him, Megan puffs and paces. "What's the difference whether my foot slipped or I hit the gas?" she argues. "Jimmy's neck is hurt. He should get something for that, right?"

Tanner is playing stone wall, but Megan can see me shrug. "Which was it?" I ask mildly.

"My foot slipped," she answers with a decisive nod, which is at once determined, defiant, and unconvincing.

"From twenty yards back?"

"Who said anything about that?"

"A witness, Megan. Someone who heard you and Jimmy argue afterward."

"Fine," she hastily backs off. "Have it your way. I rammed into him. He had another date that night. Can you believe it? Another date!"

Jimmy's face has drained to an ominous white, so I don't dare take my eyes off him. Yet I'm finally getting somewhere, and I want the rest.

"You followed him," I tell Megan. "But you didn't want him to spot you when he stopped at a light, so you stayed back. Then you got angry all over again and hit the gas. That sound about right?"

Megan shows me a little so-what shrug, and I wave my head. "And that's why you'll be getting bupkus from the Amalgamated Insurance Association of North America. You two will have to find another—more honest—way to feather your little love nest."

I can't see Megan's reaction because Jimmy has hold of my shoulders and is shaking hard.

"Listen, bitch..."

I whirl my arms inside his, chop his hands loose, and spin out of reach. When he moves in for a second grab, I kick back with my boot heel and give his shinbone a good one.

While he's still hopping, I make use of the door.

Chapter 15

The night is so thick with chilled moisture you can see it in your headlights and feel it in your flesh. I've got to crash somewhere before I literally crash, so in a moment of weakened resolve I return to Norman's. He's okay, because I see him stumbling upstairs through the front window. But either he didn't hear my knock or chose not to answer.

Just as well, really; but since I'm not willing to prostitute myself with the Lucky Leaf motel clerk, that leaves sleeping in the Taurus.

To minimize the risk, I cruise around for almost an hour searching for a neighborhood where an extra car won't automatically shout "burglar," finally choosing the driveway of a vacant house that's for sale at the end of a cul de sac. I'm warm enough curled up on the back seat under most of the clothes I packed; but the unfamiliar night noises creep me out, and I don't fall asleep sometime after midnight.

When a beat cop taps on the window, I think I've been shot.

"Do I know you?" the patrolman asks after I open the door a crack. With his flashlight beam in my face I'm sure I look like hell.

"Lauren Beck," I confess. "Used to be on the job...in my other life."

"Yeah, yeah. Thought you looked familiar. So, er, Lauren, if you don't mind my asking, what are you doing here?"

"I'm an insurance investigator now," I tell him. "I'm working."

There is a hint of dawn on the horizon, so the cop is nearing the end of his shift. He's tired and bored and cold, so he says, "Fine. You don't have to tell me what you're doing, but you can't stay here. Okay?"

"Okay," I agree.

The gym where I work out opens at five-thirty, so I drive there and catch a few more winks in the parking lot. Then I run a couple dozen laps with the pre-work crowd, shower, and dress for work. A protein drink for breakfast and I'm as ready as I'm going to get.

By now I can see that the weather has improved–for November. Flawless blue sky. A gentle breeze. The smell of fallen leaves and sun on cement. So naturally I expect to spend all morning in the office.

Two pink Post-its from David's desk are stuck to my monitor, reminding me I've neglected to set up my voicemail box. "Call me," the notes insist with Scarp's name and number underlined. The second version sports three exclamation points. I figure the homicide detective's probably worried that he can't locate his Number One suspect, but since he's not here in person brandishing handcuffs, I decide to wait a little while before getting back to him. By then maybe I'll be able prove that I had nothing to do with Corinne's death.

Sure I will. And reindeer know how to fly.

Instead, I use the landline at my desk to try to reach Garry, the cop who so recently bought me a beer at Casey's.

"Somebody's messing with me," I relate in my message, "and it might be a thug I annoyed yesterday. Can you please look into a guy named Bill Eberly, as in Eberly Electronics. Or maybe it's Bill Tanner. He's got a nephew with that last name."

Then I explain that I have no cell phone, at least until payday, "so I'll have to get back to you."

Around ten-thirty David leaves for a meeting, adding the luxury of privacy to the use of the company phone. I'll square things with my boss soon; but I figure that conversation will go better if I'm ready with an explanation.

One Mississippi, two Mississippi. A ring tone never sounded better. Then, "Eureka" a live answer.

I pour out my tale, and the wireless company's customer-relations rep speaks in that overly patient voice of a person who doesn't give a damn. "You said your cell phone was stolen along with your purse," she reports, "so we temporarily shut off your service."

"That all sounds fine except for one thing," I respond with a bit of an edge. "My purse wasn't stolen."

"Oh, good. Then you want your service reinstated, right?"

"No."

"Are you going with another carrier? Because if you are, I'm authorized to offer..."

"No!" I interrupt. "I'm calling because the woman who shut off my service wasn't me."

"It wasn't? Because whoever called had your address and account number and, and why would they...usually they just run up a huge bill. You see what I mean? Are you sure you didn't..."

"No!"

"Then who...?"

"Good question."

We agree to leave things as they are, and I hang up none the wiser.

Still no David, so I place my second call.

The VISA bank's human, when one finally comes on the line, tells me my card has been confiscated because I have a problem with my credit.

"My credit with you? Or my credit in general."

"Can't quite pin that down with what I've got, but it looks like the latter."

"So I should check with the credit agencies, is that what you're saying?" I press as Bob Battersby saunters by.

"Yes, exactly," the phone voice gladly agrees.

I slam down the receiver and set off after Bob. When I catch up with him, he's staring at David's closed door.

"Bob," I state with a huff. "Have you been messing with me?"

He turns, thrusts his lower lip forward, and blinks. "Excuse me?"

I put a foot forward and settle back on my hip. "I'd like to know whether you've been talking to Nina Wilder."

A spark lights his eyes.

"Who?"

"Nina Wilder Collins. Corinne Wilder's daughter. That would be the Corinne who just died." All of which he could have read in the newspaper.

Bob lifts his chin and contemplates my knees. "Never heard of them."

A bit late, I realize that's probably true. "How about a bad credit report? You know anything about that?"

Clasping his biceps, Battersby curls his whole body as if addressing a lower life form. "What a vivid imagination you have. Is that why David hired you? Or is this just how women work? You go around making up accusations until you accidentally learn something?"

Realizing he had a point, I copy his arm position and sigh. "Sorry. It's just that somebody's been playing some not-very-funny tricks on me, and I wondered if maybe you were hazing me, like in college." Not a great excuse, but it would have to do.

"We don't go in for that sort of thing around here," Bob responds, "but thanks for the idea."

Dumb, dumb, dumb. Not only did I give him another reason to dislike me, I'd gift-wrapped ammunition for him to use against me. *She's delusional, David. Whatever were you thinking when you hired her?*

Too embarrassed to stick around, I grab my coat and head for the elevator.

Now I'm staring at the remains of the Getaway Travel Agency, a gaping hole in the ground that smells of soggy, sooty wood and miscellaneous rubble. Metal items like file cabinets and water heaters remain, but not necessarily where they started out. Flammable material such as checkbooks and travel posters and phones are either gone or unrecognizable. Looking at the mess, I can't tell if the fire was started intentionally, but that's a determination for the experts. My job is to canvas the neighborhood for witnesses.

Turns out the only person available is the one who called the fire department, a seventy-plus woman with flashing green eyes. She's eager to talk, a little too eager. She'd been awakened by the fire's own wind and the crash of breaking windows, which means the blaze was way too far along for her to be of any help. I need a skulking figure carrying a gas can, or throwing a Molotov cocktail, something like that.

In short order I bid her good-day and head for the nearest burger joint. I've developed a pounding headache that calls for comfort food and extra-strength aspirin.

Lingering over the last of my French fries, I decide that unless I want another night in the Taurus, I'd better spend some time finding a new place to live.

Within minutes, the first Landis realtor I try concludes that my budget and her listings are incompatible. She foists me off on a company that handles semi-rural areas around Glendenning and a pert little thing with Asian features and a chipped tooth. She, at least, seems happy to meet me.

Riding around in her muddy Volvo, we begin with a Goldilocks tour of a place with ripped furniture that overlooks a grain silo. Next, a two-bedroom apartment above a tavern, and finally a small private property sandwiched between a half-finished development and a working farm. Spanning the second floor of a three-car garage, the last one-bedroom rental offers clean furniture and a little balcony with a western view. The miniscule pink bathroom is truly dreadful, but the price is right.

"I'll take it," I announce, then immediately think of Corinne. Never again will my landlord be considerate enough to let my rent to slide until my income catches up, but that's how it goes. Camelot ended, too.

Back at the roadside real estate office I sign a lease and write a deposit check. It's eighty-percent of my balance; but, again, I have no choice.

I think I better hurry up and close some cases; because if I lose my job, I'm absolutely, positively screwed.

With that thought firmly in mind I drive myself over to Jerry Shoemacher's suburban Landis two-story colonial.

The beleaguered travel agent comes off as an ordinary guy—light brown hair, medium build, brown eyes, the epitome of average, except the average person doesn't get suspected of torching his own business. Factor in some slick verve and the "Getaway" nickname and he's the perfect candidate to act in his own infomercial.

Jerry and I have been playing head games out in his sloppy, unheated garage for fifteen minutes, either because he lies better with something in his hands, or because his horoscope told him November 14 was the cosmic deadline for winterizing one's lawnmower. I don't know about him, but I'm ready for a break.

"May I please borrow your phone?" I beg. "It's local." I'm dying to know if the landlord gave me the apartment.

Jerry balks before he remembers that he needs my good will. Then he makes like a gracious host and leads me inside.

"What!" I yell when Chris-with-the-chipped-tooth delivers the bad news. "Insufficient funds." My check bounced.

No deposit. No apartment.

I desperately want to scream, but I just spin around and mouth a bad word. When I settle back into my skin, I notice the travel agent's open-mouthed stare.

"Gotta go," I announce, already hurrying out the door and down the driveway.

"Will this hold up my claim?" Jerry shouts at my back.

Chapter 16

The branch of the First Federal Bank of Glendenning nearest my former home sits on the corner of Susquehanna and Fourth like a gray stone crypt. On the rare occasion when I go inside, I always get a big hello from an assistant manager named Dennis Arquette. So it is he I am hoping to see when I trot past the purple and white decorative cabbages and push through the rear double doors.

Dennis smiles over the head of the bald man in his customer chair, so I point at the two upholstered love seats bracketed by brass railing to indicate that I'm willing to wait.

Yet before I sit down my attention is drawn to the other end of the room. A woman who's been working a promotional table is clearing up a continental breakfast. Used to be I wouldn't have noticed her let alone approached, but today? I saunter over.

"Whatcha got here?"

"The bank is offering a new money-management plan. The coffee and donuts were for customers who came in to hear about it." Her blonde hair is a perfectly sprayed mound, and her fitted jacket is garnished with a silk gardenia.

"But you seem to be done now," I observe, "so do you mind? I missed breakfast, and I've got to wait for Dennis to finish with that man over there, and then..." During this cheeky blather I'm filling a cardboard cup with black decaf and setting two crullers on a napkin.

The bank salesperson is taken aback, to say the least. I'm well dressed, if you discount the wrinkles, so I don't

look like the type to cadge coffee and donuts. Yet that's
what I seem to be doing, and Miscellaneous here wants to
rap my knuckles with a ruler.

"But…" she begins her protest.

"They're the bank's donuts, right? And the bank's
coffee?"

"Well, yes."

"And I'm a bank customer. So thanks. It's awfully nice
of you to share."

Back at the waiting area I set my cardboard cup on a
magazine with shaking fingers and spread the napkin with
the crullers on my lap. I worry that the food won't go down
my throat, but then I remember I'm homeless and low on
cash, my credit is shot, and I have no phone.

The crullers taste like dirt, the coffee like tar, but I
persevere. The amplified remarks of people in their cars
and the tellers' replies offer background noise while the
clock hands slowly tick forward. Doors open and close as
customers do their business and leave. No one appears to
notice that I'm not the same Lauren Beck who arrived only
minutes ago.

No point in denying that I feel violated and annoyed—
alright, *pissed*—by everything that's been going on, but
I've kept a lid on my anger because what I've lost are
external things, conveniences I've convinced myself I can
live without.

This morning's development blows the lid right off.
Finessing food—essentially stealing it in broad daylight—
degrades me in a way I can neither ignore nor tolerate.
Enough is enough. Whoever is after me had better turn and
run, because now I'm coming after them.

The decision straightens my back and swells my lungs.
I feel whole again. For the life of me I can't imagine why
the turnaround took so long.

Actually, that isn't quite true. Nina is the reason. Deep down I've always known that she was threatened by my close relationship with her mother. Corinne and I had so much in common--cancer, my father, music, and more. Nina always resented that, just as I've always regretted making her feel left out; and because I suspect she might be behind the dirty tricks, I've hesitated to retaliate.

This morning changed all that. This morning exceeded my limit. If I find out Nina has been waging a secret vendetta, she had better brace herself for battle.

"You've got sugar on your lip," Dennis remarks when his visitor's chair is finally mine.

"Thanks," I tell him, wiping the powder off with my wrist.

"Now, what can I do for you?" His square, open face is sallow, and he's done that self-delusional thing with strands of hair across his head. Still, his lips curve into the most welcoming smile I've ever seen.

"I need to understand why one of my checks bounced."

While his computer accesses my account, the banker mentions a road rally being held in New Jersey over the weekend. "I could pair you up if you're interested." He saw my Miata at the drive-up window a couple years ago and has been trying to recruit me into his hobby ever since.

I wave my head. "Not a good week for me, Den."

The assistant manager's smile doesn't flicker. "Okay," he says, already focusing on his screen. "What's going on here?"

"I put a down-payment on an apartment. It should have cleared, but it didn't."

"Guess you spent more on that trip than you thought."

Oh, please. Not again. "What trip?" I ask.

"The trip you called about the other week. You said you lost your debit card and asked us to overnight you a new one. I figured since you were such a long-time customer..."

"Shit."

"I beg your pardon?"

"Sorry." I hastily explain about the opened mail, the tampering with my credit and the cell phone.

"Identity theft," he murmurs as if that explains everything.

"No," I argue, although I don't blame him for getting it wrong. "It's just theft."

Dennis looks as blank as you might expect. "What's the difference?"

Once again, the difference is the cell phone. The culprit isn't some opportunistic crook taking me for what little I'm worth. Suspending my wireless service profits nobody. All it does is harass me, which suggests that the motive is personal.

Still, the distinction won't mean a thing to Dennis.

"What's left in my checking account?" I inquire.

"Seventy-nine thirty seven."

It should be nine hundred and change, enough to cover the apartment deposit.

"Okay. How about we just close this sucker out and start over?"

Dennis shakes his head. "That'll take a couple of weeks. Time for any outstanding checks to clear."

"But there's just the one that bounced." I show him my checkbook to prove it, but the banker holds firm.

Inside I'm bursting, but I make an heroic effort to sound calm. "The impostor ordered a new debit card, right?"

"Right."

"How? By phone?"

"No. We require a signature. She went to the Green Street branch, and they called us for permission."

"You the one who gave it?"

Dennis's face floods with color. "Green Street told me you were going on a trip in two days, and that you couldn't find your debit card."

"What about the PIN number?" All anyone needs to get cash out of my checking account. No signature, just punch in a couple of anonymous numbers.

"Changed."

"Because you believed my card had been lost. And, of course, I changed my mailing address because...?"

Dennis's thumbs are now hooked behind his belt. "You moved," he says. "The card went to a post office box."

He sits forward in his chair and spreads his hands. "The woman knew your mother's maiden name, Lauren. I had no reason to suspect she wasn't you."

I argue that point, with apparent success, because half an hour later I leave with sixty-eight dollars and fifteen cents, the checkbook balance minus fees. Dennis looks miserable. I am miserable.

Only one of the five employees at the Green Street branch remembers my name, but she can't describe my impersonator.

Indeed, everyone there seems to regard me as a nuisance and a quack, possibly, just *possibly*, because of my attitude. So I figure why not fulfill their expectations? I stride to the middle of the lobby, cup my hands around my mouth, and yell, "You'll be hearing from my lawyer!"

Other than a few appalled customers, only two people allow themselves to meet my eyes, a manager and the armed guard, and he steps toward me with his hand on the butt of his gun.

He also follows me out and watches me drive away.

Chapter 17

After making a scene at the Green Street branch of my bank, I need a place to sit and think; so I drive to a Clemens Supermarket, park next to a cart shed, and shut off the engine. At three-thirty on a Friday afternoon nobody will give me a second glance.

Lists are wonderful. Lists make your priorities beautifully clear. Food, clothing—like that. Safety comes first; no more sleeping in the car. Driving myself to a Philadelphia homeless shelter is an insane idea, and I wouldn't take a bed from a battered woman for the world. The AIA office might—*might*—work. Although I'm not sure how I would explain myself tonight to the guard.

So, since dignity is a luxury I can no longer afford, my list reads "Joseph, Wilma, Melanie, and George." They are, respectively, my hairdresser, my dry cleaner, a sort of a former high-school friend who is half-owner of a baby-clothes shop, and Corinne's mailman. I consider George to be a last resort; he's a terrible grouch, and if I were to miss him at the post office, I wouldn't have a clue where else to look.

Before I lose my nerve, I back out of the parking space and head for Joseph's beauty "emporium," which is in a strip mall outside Landis next to a bagel bakery.

Overlooking my somber expression, my hairdresser tosses out his typical "Come to get your lettuce chopped?" greeting while teasing white hair into an arc over a thin-lipped woman's eye.

"Not this time," I reply.

"Good, because I know you don't have an appointment; and as you can see, I'm up to my ass in alligator pumps."

One client has just arrived, one is reading *Vogue* under a dome dryer, and another with a head full of pointy dark-brown spikes waits out the dye-timer by filing her nails.

No choice, I remind myself. "Speak to you a minute?"

Joseph stops in mid-primp to stare at me. His receding butch cut, his black-rimmed glasses, indeed his whole head is bracketed by his long, graceful fingers.

"Something's wrong," he states. "You're allergic, aren't you? I knew it. You can't just put chemicals on yourself forever, you know. The body's bound to rebel." Joseph lifts his eyes in a brief homage to the gods then returns to his comb-out.

The "chemical" comment refers to my blonde highlights. "No, I'm not allergic. Nothing's the matter with me at all. No, that's not true. A lot's the matter." I sigh with exasperation. "Can you just give me a minute? Please?"

This isn't part of Joseph's daily script. While he hesitates, the white-haired lady swivels her head to show me how irritated she is.

"You're done," I tell her. "Why don't you just leave your money on the counter?"

Joseph has barely enough time to remove the plastic drape before she scooches out of the chair. She huffs as she stomps away.

Behind me a timer buzzes. "I better..." The hair stylist gives an all encompassing wave.

"In a second," I interject. "Can I stay with you tonight?"

If there were no audience and more time, I might have cushioned that with an explanation, but Joseph's horrified expression tells me his answer would have been the same.

"No," he says. "I can't believe you asked."

"Me either," I state honestly.

"Make an appointment," he calls after me. "You're looking pretty shaggy."

TLC Dry Cleaning is located to the left of a farmer's market where Corinne and I often shop. Shopped. I still can't accept that she's gone.

Wilma, the proprietor, rings up a customer as I enter. She is a short, soft-bodied woman well over fifty clothed in a gray skirt and lavender sweater set. Lavender buttons, not pearl; and as always she wears laced black shoes and support hose. A few years ago we were making idle conversation about THE DaVINCI CODE while she collected my clothes. Her observations were both astute and funny, and I realized that her shy exterior concealed a clever and discerning mind. I told her so, and we've been book friends ever since.

"Hi," I greet her, after the jingle bells on the door quit ringing.

The vestibule smells of warm fabric and hot metal. Wilma once boasted that the moving overhead racks have been in regular use since the sixties with only two repairs, which caused me to notice that they were fuzzy with lint-covered oil. In spite of my security lecture, sunlight still steals in through a half-opened door in the back; but, as Wilma pointed out, "people gotta breathe."

And eat.

And sleep.

Perhaps I should also mention that Wilma is reticent in a distrustful, old-world way I don't pretend to understand. Perhaps because of that, conversing with her makes me feel giddy, as if I've been singled out for the honor of hearing her voice. Already, I feel that way now.

Because my hands are empty and she knows I'm not here for a pick-up, she lifts a black, badly penciled eyebrow.

We are alone, so this is the perfect time to speak; yet when I open my mouth only air comes out. All I can l think of is me in those black lace-ups listening to a plea for shelter from a customer who doesn't even know my last name.

"Never mind," I say, pivoting on my heel.

Next on the list is Melanie Fox, but I decide against going there. She and I like to think we've outgrown our high-school differences; we've even done lunch twice to congratulate ourselves on how nicely we've evolved. However, she has a husband and two kids, and I realize it's foolhardy to even consider putting any of them at risk.

Since George the Mailman was a farcical notion from the start, that about does it for my list.

The Taurus's dashboard clock reads five-twenty; but it's Friday, so the bank will still be open. I find Dennis Arquette totally absorbed by his computer.

"I need your help, Dennis," I blurt. "Really, truly, honestly need your help. Not the bank's—yours."

He turns from the screen to offer me a couple of blinks. "Me?" It's Dennis the person now, not Dennis the mid-level manager. Sensing my angst, a little empathetic sweat has formed in the creases of his forehead.

"Yes, you." Editing out the murder accusation, I briefly list my problems, concluding with, "I have no place to sleep tonight, Dennis. Also, I have nobody else to ask. So I'm asking you. May I sleep on your sofa tonight? Please take some time to think about your answer, because it's either your place or risk getting raped in my car."

I can actually hear him gulp.

"Er, yes. I guess so. Okay."

Unbeknownst to me, Dennis lives in Colmar with his adult daughter, Janice. Within thirty seconds of his agreeing to house me for the night, the assistant bank manager is on the phone trying to explain me to her. An obvious omission is my gender, which I completely understand. Middle-aged men don't usually bring home women they scarcely know, not in suburban Philadelphia anyway.

"I hope you like corned beef and cabbage," he remarks after he hangs up the phone.

"Yes, sure. Of course," I gush. "I'll be glad for anything."

He nods once then returns to his work, reminding me that dinner will not be ours for quite a while.

I don't dare leave and come back, so I watch each customer as if they're here to stab me in the back or at least steal my purse.

Meanwhile, Dennis is glancing at me less and less but with more and more concern. Occasionally he ducks into the safe-deposit vault to service a customer, and once he excuses himself to go to the employees' lounge. I'm pleased to learn where that is. It's awkward enough hogging a visitor's chair for hours on end; I prefer not to invite more interest by inquiring about a rest room.

"You'll follow me?" he remarks when at last the bank has closed and we've emerged into the parking lot together. In the light spreading from the upper corners of the bank I see that my benefactor is a man transformed--deflated, as if work was his stage, and with the curtain down he can return to being a natural introvert. Even more he resembles an undertaker or perhaps the man in the "American Gothic" painting, and not for the first time I wonder what I've gotten myself into.

"Gotta pick up a toothbrush," I lie. "Why don't you just give me directions?" For all I know we're being monitored by the wrong people as we speak, so for the Arquette's sake I intend to use an evasive route.

Dennis hesitates, but complies; and as soon as his car carefully slips onto Main Street, it hits me. I've got an unknown enemy, and I've attached myself to a stranger.

Nevertheless, I perform my lengthy roundabout drive and park half-block away from the Arquette's door. One of several similar houses on the tree-lined street, their home is a tall old dame with a full-sized porch and two overgrown evergreens dominating the front lawn.

A late-thirties woman who has the misfortune to resemble her dad answers my knock , and Dennis rises from an ornate pink sofa to introduce us.

"Janice, this is Lauren Beck. Lauren, this is my daughter, Janice Arquette."

"Hello," she says, offering me the fingertips of her right hand. They feel hot, as if her nervous system is easily disturbed and I've caused a flare-up.

"You'll use my room," my host offers. "I've asked Janice to freshen the sheets."

"No, really," I protest. "That isn't necessary. The sofa will be fine."

"Yes, it will. Fine for me."

"Shall we sit down to dinner?" the daughter suggests.

"By all means." My stomach is already dancing with anticipation.

A second room jammed with dark Victorian furnishings suggests that some long-gone woman favored lace curtains, delicate ceramics, and pink. Flowered paper stifles every wall, and tucked behind a ten-inch cross bearing the Christ figure depicted in gold is a folded strip of palm leaf so dry and brittle it no longer possesses color. All in all the polar opposite of Norman's casual, welcoming home.

Janice and I sit on either side of the dining room table, her father between us at the end. Holding hands for a solemn blessing further underscores how thoroughly I've invaded their lives, and my discomfort nears the level of pain.

The Arquette's faces glow when at last they raise their eyes.

I hasten to break the spell. "So, Janice. Do you work outside of the home?" Perhaps not the most delicate way of getting to know another woman, but right now it's all I've got.

Father and daughter exchange a glance. "Jan is an electrical engineer," Dennis answers. "A very good one, too."

"How interesting," I remark. And it is. I can easily see this sturdy woman doing something mathematical and bright, something involving precision that doesn't rely much on people skills.

"How about you?" She has passed me the tureen containing meat, cabbage and potatoes, so I serve myself as I deliver my reply.

"Used to be a cop, then computer research. Now I'm an insurance investigator."

"Oh!" Jan exclaims, her face brightening. "So that's why you're in trouble. I thought it had something to do with a man."

Dennis barks a disapproving, "Jan!" but she waves it away.

"Oh come on, Dad. You were thinking that too."

His sudden blush is a signed confession.

In the quiet our knives and forks might as well be bulldozers and chain saws.

"I imagine what you're dealing with is quite confidential," Dennis hints.

I nearly choke on a piece of potato. Could he really be sparing me an explanation, trusting me entirely on faith? I'm not even sure it's safe for them to remain so completely in the dark, yet that is clearly their preference.

Father and daughter await my answer.

"Yes," I respond, and the tableau is broken.

After the housekeeping chores are completed and I'm alone in Dennis's bedroom, I lock the door, jam a chair under the knob, and shudder.

Chapter 18

Saturday breakfast at the Arquette residence is lavish and early. Fresh-baked biscuits and jam, scrambled eggs, sausage, and home fries. The coffee has chicory in it, which I hate, but I compliment Janice on it anyway and force it down. Food is not to be taken for granted.

"Well," I say, as my breakfast petrifies in my stomach. "You've both been extremely kind, and I can't thank you enough, but I've got to get going." I push away from the table, pleased that I had the foresight to leave my duffle by the door.

"Bye," I wave as both my hosts stand holding their breath.

Yet less than a minute later I'm back, my jaw clenched to keep from swearing.

"Yes?" Dennis inquires, his distress hard to miss.

"Flat tires," I am forced to report. "Four of them."

The tires might or might not be ruined, I'll find out later; I'm too eager to get myself away from the Arquettes.

"You have any vindictive neighbors?" I quiz Dennis during the drive to pick up my Miata. The side trip will make him late for work; but if getting rid of me means mushing through Alaska, he's ready to hire a dog sled.

He shrugs before tossing out an answer. "Earl Schneider has a bit of a temper."

"Am I parked in front of his house?"

"Not really."

"Whose house *am* I in front of?"

"Polly and Paul Linton. They have three kids and a dog.

Polly'll have to carry groceries a little farther, but I doubt either of them would have done that to your car."

"How about the kids?"

"The oldest is ten."

I'll phone the Lintons to ask if they saw anything and to apologize for leaving the Taurus there until Monday, but Dennis puts the thought out of my head by pulling into my old driveway before I can ask to be dropped at the curb. I didn't want Nina to notice anything until I had the Miata fired up and in gear.

Too late now. The kitchen curtain just moved.

What the hell. Be nice to pick up some more clothes. I thank Dennis for the fourth time, and stroll up to the house.

Arms folded, Corinne's daughter stands just inside the kitchen door looking stony-faced but not exactly knife-in-my-gut hostile, which I view as a progress of sorts.

However, it's soon clear that she has no intention of letting me in; so, foolish as it feels, I dig out my keys and unlock the door.

It opens about twelve inches before encountering Nina's foot.

"Excuse me," I say, slithering around her. Our shoulders bump, but she maintains her hardened stare. *Fine*, I think to myself. *Be that way.* "I'm getting more of my stuff."

Jilly is watching Animal Planet and eating a sliced apple. "Hey, girlfriend," I greet her.

"Hey," she replies with a bashful smile.

"How's Cousteau?" I ask.

"Fine."

"Any trouble?" I lift my chin half an inch toward Nina, who's making noise back in the laundry room.

Negative. "He's in my room. Don't unplug him until you have to."

"Okay."

I can't help myself, I look into the girl's bedroom on my way past.

Swimmie's tank sits on a sturdy-looking desk next to some polka dot folders and a box of magic markers. Added to his sleeping castle are a cluster of plastic palm trees and a toy treasure chest overflowing with pretend doubloons. Depending on which direction he chooses to face, he has a panoramic view of the outdoors or of Jilly doing homework. The fish net I use whenever I need to freshen his water waits on the windowsill in a tall blue sand bucket.

"Hi, Mom. I'm home," gets as far as the tip of my tongue, but the old routine suddenly seems silly and stale.

With the fish looking on I borrow Jilly's purple marker and a sheet of notebook paper.

"He's yours," I write. "Love, Lauren." Then I blow my former roommate a final kiss and take myself on out of there.

Other than the missing fish tank, my place looks the same.

No, that isn't strictly true. It looks wilted, as if I dropped my clean clothes on the wicker sofa two years ago instead of last week. It smells close, too, as if the attic ghosts have already reclaimed their turf.

I shove aside my flowered comforter and sit on the edge of the bed. Look around. All this stuff is just stuff, I remind myself, and inanimate objects stopped mattering to me some time ago.

Plenty of other things to think about though, so I just sit and wait for the conflicting sensations to sort themselves out.

I've never had a week like this one, not even when I was battling cancer. Then at least I knew what I was up against—a random act of nature. Nothing personal, Lauren, but here's your very own life-threatening test. Go, girl.

This isn't like that.

Corinne knew that I'd won the war but was still fighting the battle. Wise woman that she was, she patiently waited for me to rebuild my confidence. When she sensed it was time, she encouraged me to apply for the AIA job. Her recommendations had always been on target before; so if she thought I was ready, I trusted her judgment. Now I can't help wondering how much Nina's welfare factored into Corinne's final advice.

And what about turning down my dad? I still don't get that.

But these are two troubling thoughts I can examine later. Right now I just want to slip away and take a break from it all.

I find my old gym bag and stuff it with clothes and toiletries, a shopping bag and load it with shoes. The Miata's trunk is challenged, but I slam it shut and hop behind the wheel.

I'm going where everybody goes when they're down and out, to the people who will take me in no matter what. Dad lives in Albuquerque, my brother in Maryland, so Ron wins on simple arithmetic.

To shorten the drive I put in an oldies CD, bittersweet nostalgia from the childhood of rock 'n roll.

"I wants to walk you home," Fats Domino croons as I shift into drive and hit the gas.

Chapter 19

My father thinks he and his son get along just fine; my brother thinks my father is full of it. They're both right. They just labor under the masculine delusion that commenting on baseball, or basketball or junior women's bowling is the same as communicating. I know different. I know they've only ever had two things in common, genetics and farming; and after Dad began to dabble in real estate, farming became a sore issue.

I contemplate this as I speed down the nicely landscaped Blue Route, Pennsylvania's 476, toward I-95 south, where I switch to worrying about sleepy truck drivers overlooking my small red sports car.

After I pass the "Welcome to Maryland" sign, I change subjects again, this time to my brother and me. In twenty minutes I will arrive at Ronnie's new farm–best to be emotionally prepared.

How to put this? Ron and I don't even talk about sports. Somehow during the four years before my birth he got the notion that he would be an only child, so right away I impacted his self-image. If he'd been good enough, loveable enough, or just plain *enough*, Mom and Dad wouldn't have had me.

Later, when he discovered I didn't play like a boy, look like a boy, or speak like a boy, I became that loathsome liability, a little sister.

It got better, and then it got worse. Ronnie went to agricultural college and came home expecting to work the family farm alongside Dad until he had sons of his own to work beside him. He loved our farm, not the way you love

a sunset or a comfortable pair of loafers. He loved the soil
the way you and I love oxygen. The precious, precarious
life cycles of the flora and fauna around him continue to be
all the drama his life requires. I envied him that, knowing
himself from the get-go and never wavering from his goals.

Yet if our dad sensed the depth of Ron's attachment to
the Glendenning homestead, he never acknowledged it.
Like Corinne, my father is more pragmatic than romantic.
Farming doesn't pay? Fine, let's try selling land. Woman
turns you down? Checkout the southwest. Marry a potter
you just met? Sure, why not?

As I exit onto a two-lane road studded with white
wooden cottages, Fats Domino finishes his set and waves
on K. D. Lang. Sweet stuff, and restful, too, in the way that
the ensuing countryside calms me—open space suddenly
divided by a stand of trees, brief folksy towns that sell
crafts and crabs, forests full of small houses, vacation
homes gathered beside estuaries and rivers and ultimately
the Chesapeake Bay. Maryland is a floating leaf with a
hundred pointy lobes—anywhere you go, you almost
always encounter water.

Ron owns a hundred and ten acres inland and rents
twenty more. Small by farm standards; but I feel sure he'll
increase his holdings or die trying. Turning into the long
gravel lane, it amazes me how much his place reminds me
of home. Maybe the brick house is a little too modern, but
the fallow fields and the barn and the various sheds and
cribs are right out of Childhood 101.

Karen, Ron's wife, emerges from the kitchen before I
brake to a stop, the advantage of a half-mile lane—you
always know who's coming. Appearing to be pleasantly
surprised, she saunters over to the car.

"Lauren," she says, wrapping me in a long-armed hug.
She's tall, taller than Ron truth be told, and much blonder

than me. A fair-skinned, straight-down-her-back, yellow-haired Norwegian with the requisite cornflower blue eyes. Her two daughters are Xerox copies. Aged six and seven, they're jostling through the front door in puffy pastel jackets.

Ron finishes ushering the girls outside before nodding hello. "Lauren," he remarks, his surprise more of the Now-what? variety. "We were just going out."

"Not a problem," I assure him. "Just wanted to see you, that's all."

That isn't all, and he knows it. So does Karen. I've never arrived unannounced before, and my last visit was Christmas—eleven months ago.

"I heard about Corinne," Karen sympathizes. "I'm so sorry."

"Thanks." They've been speaking to Daddy I realize, stifling an unwarranted pang of jealousy.

The reminder served to soften Ron's attitude. Arresting features and a farmer's hard body caused my brother to become a swaggering, swearing youth then an extremely sensitive young adult. Karen cured him of most of the macho bullshit, but I'm sure my brother still considers himself to be a man's man.

"We were getting ready to run some errands," he tells me now. "You want coffee or something while...?"

"Yeah, sure."

"Or you could come along..."

Karen has let Ron be Ron long enough. She grabs my shoulder and wiggles it twice before playfully pushing me toward the front door. "Why don't you and the girls get going," she tells her husband. "Lauren and I will be fine until you come back. Right, Lauren?"

"Right." It is Karen, I realize, I've been most eager to see. She's honest to the point of brutal bluntness, a quality I happen to admire. She also has a rounded nose you're tempted to discount and broad, flat cheeks that enhance her eyes, eyes that are intent upon watching you.

"Coffee and crumb cake?" she offers, steering me past their earthy Scandinavian-style living area into the kitchen.

"Yours?" I ask, my mouth already watering.

"Sara Lee's. Who has time?"

"I'll forgive you for not baking if you give me an extra big slice."

While Karen gathers our coffee and cake, I wait on the padded stool of a breakfast bar facing a huge picture window. The view encompasses a white-gray dome of sky and a plowed-over field that skirts to within ten feet of the house—my efficient brother getting the most out of the land. Close by several English sparrows with shadows black as puddles peck at whatever they can find in the mud.

By the time my sister-in-law settles down beside me, my face is smeared with tears.

It takes a minute or two, but I finally turn toward her. Her expression says what it needs to.

"He didn't come to the funeral," I confide. "He didn't even raise a glass to her like he was supposed to."

"Your dad."

"Yes, my dad. I'm beginning to think I don't even know him."

"What gives you that impression?"

"He told me Corinne didn't want him spending money to come East if..."

"You mean when."

"Okay, when. But she told him to put some of their music on and raise a glass to her; and when I asked if he'd done it, he said, "Not yet.""

Karen takes a deep breath and checks on the sparrows before she responds. "You know Annie's a recovering alcoholic, right?"

My own lungs seem to collapse. I can scarcely bark out the word no.

Ron's wife merely nods. "So what else is going on? Surely you didn't come here just to complain about your father. That you could have done on the phone."

I'm thinking, *not really,* and the craziness of that makes me laugh, just a little sardonic snort.

Karen's blue eyes widen. "Now I'm really curious," she says.

I claw at my hair and release another nervous laugh. "I'm homeless," I confess with a feint of my head. "Nina tossed me out, and I can't pay for another place right now."

My sister-in-law becomes so still that I hold my breath, too. "You'll stay here," she finally states, spanking the table as if it were a done deal.

I resume breathing, surprised by the extent of my relief. "I'd like to. For a few days at least, if Ron doesn't mind."

"He'll come around," she says with a mischievous wink.

The two of us regard each other for a moment. Then I take a sip of coffee while Karen remains pensive, as if she has something more to say.

"He doesn't blame you, you know," she remarks when the time finally comes. "Not really."

I haven't come here to talk about that, so I wave her off. "Don't worry about it. It doesn't matter."

"Of course it matters. You deserved to go to college. Ron did, so why not you? Then the cancer!" She makes a disgusted tsk. "Who could have predicted that? No, Charlie would have had to sell off those parcels anyway. How else was he going to retire?"

I shake my head. "I don't fault Ron for feeling cheated. He loved that farm. If I could get it back and give it to him now, I would."

Karen slaps her knee. "Yeah, me, too. But that ain't likely. We're doing fine, Sis. Don't you give it a second thought."

Tell that to Ronnie, I want to say; but I know it won't help. I love my brother, but his self-examinations are as short and shallow as his morning shave. I steer the conversation to what Karen and the kids had been up to; and when the coffee is gone, I ask to borrow their phone.

Karen crosses the room to load the dishwasher, and I get the number of the Paul Linton family from Directory Assistance. When a woman answers, I tell her my name.

"It's my company car with the four flat tires in front of your house," I explain. "I hope you don't mind if I wait until Monday to get it towed. It's a new job for me, and I'm not sure how to handle repair problems yet."

"Wait a minute. You say it's your car?"

"Yes. Why do you ask?"

"Because this guy...you're sure it's yours?"

"Well, yeah." A chill of dread snakes up my spine. Nina enticing a man to break the law for her is unimaginable; she had enough trouble recruiting two male acquaintances to help her move. "I'll show you the owner's card on Monday; but please, you said something about a man."

I hear a chair scrape and an intake of breath. "It was pretty weird, really," Mrs. Linton begins. "First a cop knocked on our door and told us the car was stolen. He wanted to know if we saw who parked it out front."

"That would have been me."

"Oh, yeah?"

"I was visiting the Arquettes."

"Wow! That's really spooky, because my husband was standing right there when the cop phoned whoever made the complaint."

"Any idea what was said?"

"Oh, yeah. The guy told the cop it was all a big mistake, that his nephew snitched the keys to his company car, something like that. Then he said the kid had learned his lesson, and he refused to press charges. Made the cop so furious he told the guy he was on his own picking it up. Then this morning—all those flat tires—wow! You don't think the cop...?"

I tell her I doubt very much that the cop slashed my tires. "Did you or your husband notice anybody strange hanging around the neighborhood last night?"

"Sorry. The both of us go to bed kinda early, what with the kids and all."

The room around me has grown steadily smaller until now it feels like the inside of a trash compactor. Tricking the police into finding me—Wow! as Mrs. Linton likes to say. That was big. Desperate and gutsy, and very very scary. A warning in more ways than one. Enough to make a person sleep lightly and watch her back all day.

Karen stops drying a pot with a dishtowel and asks what's wrong.

"Long story."

"But you'll explain later, right?" Ronnie and the two girls have just burst in rattling shopping bags and clamoring for their lunch.

"Sure," I reply, but my mind is already on something else.

Like how easy it would be to follow a rusty red convertible.

Chapter 20

Since kids and interruptions go together like ham and cheese, the details of my plight emerged in bits and pieces throughout the weekend. Karen handled everything from the potato-chip squabble to the broken bicycle with patience and humor, but what I appreciated most was how welcome she made me feel. This was the home life I almost forgot existed.

For example Saturday night. Dinner here is an occasion—candles, a special meal. No squabbling allowed, and no TV. Trying to be a good guest, I joked about the on-the-job mistakes I'd made so far—fibbing to get the goods on the old golfer, giving Jimmy Tanner a flat tire and then getting chased. Karen started laughing right away, but it wasn't until I described Electronics Thug's bologna breath that Ronnie hid his mouth behind a calloused hand and joined in. Watching their father, the two girls giggled, too, and finally—finally—seemed to warm toward me.

This morning I helped make German potato salad in advance of dinner. I folded laundry and threw in a load of my own. Now it's Sunday afternoon, and young Terry and I just lost the fourth hand of Go Fish to Charlene.

My brother, who rarely relaxes, is slouched on the sofa reading the paper and listening to the Redskins game on TV. In a chair over by a floor lamp, Karen glances up from her crewel work to marvel at him.

"So, Sis," Ron opens with an exaggerated ease, "you want a tour of the farm?"

I perk right up. "Love it."

"I'll finish your card game," Karen offers with a conspiratorial grin. "Use my sheepskin jacket. It's on the hook."

Crunching across the driveway gravel, Ron takes it for granted that I'll keep up or risk being left behind, an old habit of his; and at long last I match him stride for stride. When we get to what looks like an enormous Quonset hut, he unlatches a human-sized door and gestures me inside.

"This is the barn," he says.

"Oh, really?" Stepping into the muddy aisle of stalls, the odors of warm animals, hay, and fresh manure transport me back twenty years.

"Always the wise ass," my brother observes. "Probably why you're in so much trouble." His crooked smile tilts his dark blond mustache and dimples his left cheek. He has acquired crow's feet, I notice, and a few strands of gray mingle with his light brown hair. I think he looks terrific.

"In here," he says, opening another door to the right.

"I see you finally cleaned your room."

We've entered a heated, surprisingly neat office complete with a copier-fax-printer and a spanking new computer. Shelves full of ring binders, equipment catalogs, and breeding books line the inner wall. A table holds cardboard boxes of broken harnesses and other whatnot needing attention, and to my right two mullioned windows overlook a muddy fenced area. In June the corral will be ringed with fragrant grass, maybe even daisies. Now it is fringed with dry brown stubble.

Ron rests his foot on a bench, leans on his knee and gestures me toward the nearest seat. Tour over. Big brother wants to talk.

My chair is a dented gray metal thing so cold and hard it makes me want to sit on my hands, but I'm afraid it'll be hot enough soon.

"You told Karen you're homeless," my brother reports. "Was that some sort of joke?"

"I wish."

Ron lifts an eyebrow. Then he sinks onto the bench, rests his forearms on his splayed legs, and gives me a heavy sigh. "Lauren, Lauren, Lauren," he laments with a sad wave of his head.

I haven't been alone with my sibling in years; and it feels odd, as if we've just met. This man, this handsome man, is my *brother*—not my rival or tormentor or any of the obsolete labels I formerly used to justify avoiding him.

Then he says, "Let's hear it," in our father's voice, and something in my chest rips open. I launch into, "Nina wants to believe I euthanized Corinne because I couldn't stand her suffering...," and I don't stop until Ron has heard it all. Everything—from the opened mail to the four slashed tires.

Listening, my brother's face grows more and more grave. "So why aren't you dead?" he asks so bluntly I have to laugh.

"Because I'm a Beck?" By reputation, Beck chickens are too tough to eat.

"That was a serious question, L.L.," for Lauren Louise, as the close to an endearment as Ron ever gets.

"I know, I know," I say. "And it's a good one. But I just can't seem to get my head around it, you know?"

My brother waits in silence, the same way our Dad always forced us to concentrate; and after a minute and a couple of deep breaths, I address the problem for real.

"It's an amateur..." I begin. Being new at the work, David has only given me cases perpetrated by lightweights.

"Likely," Ron agrees with a nod, "considering that's who you've been annoying lately. But...?"

"But I guess I'm still alive because the perp doesn't want me dead." To a clever, determined killer murder is disturbingly easy. Nearly impossible to prevent, in fact.

"Go on."

"Nobody else to frame..."

Ron nods. "... for Corinne," he finishes for me. It's unlikely that Nina killed her mother; but if she did, I was the only available scapegoat.

"What else?"

"Or else discrediting me is enough." *For now*, I realize.

"How do you figure?"

"Say it's Bob Battersby, the asshole at work. You ever hear that name?"

"No."

"So probably no Beck connection, right?"

Ron shrugs.

"So probably all he wants is for me to get fired or quit. Getting violent would be overkill. Messy, risky—ridiculous!"

"Okay."

"If it's Megan and Jimmy, they might think getting my work reassigned would give them another shot at the jackpot—or maybe they just get off on petty revenge. Who knows?"

Ron waffles his hand back and forth. "Revenge sounds more like it, but the pivotal word is 'petty.' So far, you've just been a pain in the ass—nothing new. Which is why I'm surprised the dirtbag's gone to so much trouble."

I smile as the knee-jerk little-sister mechanism kicks in. "You still think I can't take care of myself?" I once flipped him to the ground because he didn't believe I could.

"Hell, no," my brother replies with a shake of his head. "I'm worried about the sleezeball." He flexes his shoulders and rubs his palms along his pant legs, and that's it. End of moment.

I stand and massage my butt with both hands—that's one hell of an unforgiving chair—then right away realize I've left something out. Part of a sentence, half of a thought. A second later it clicks.

"Hey, bro," I say, easing into my request. "Borrow your computer?"

"Sure." He rises to leave. "But don't be late for dinner. Karen's a bear when her biscuits get cold."

"I'll bet."

"I'm not kidding. It isn't pretty."

Other brothers and sisters might have hugged about then, but not us. Ron just slides a rolling desk chair under my unhappy butt, gives me a little smile from the doorway and poof, he's gone. I listen to his footsteps until they're less than a whisper, then I snap out of it.

Signing onto Ron's access company as a guest, I go to the site for the *Glendenning Daily News.*

"Open says me," I murmur, dredging up the silly childhood play on words.

An instant later I type the phrase most likely to summon the information I want. Then I limit the search to the past fourteen days and hit "enter."

"Whatdya know," I marvel over the fourth hit on the list. "Eberly Electronics got robbed."

And guess who took pictures.

Chapter 21

The fact that suspected murderers aren't supposed to leave the state had conveniently slipped my mind; so after shutting down my brother's computer, I use the last few minutes before dinner to call Scarp's cell phone from the privacy of Ron's office. No answer, though, so I apologize to the homicide detective's voice-mail, adding that I'm at my brother's in Maryland and will be back at work on Monday.

Then, based on the fuss made by the men loading the truck, I mention that I might have digital shots of the Eberly robbery taking place and will e-mail them from the AIA office. Robbery isn't Scarp's bailiwick, but he'll know where to forward the information.

When I return to the house, Karen glances up from the oven with an mischievous smile.

"What?" I ask.

"We've got a surprise for you," she can't wait to confess.

I am to borrow her cell phone, credit card, and car. When I protest—mildly, I admit—she flicks blonde hair over her shoulder and kids that she'll be good for the Miata's image.

Ron puts it another way. "Oh, you'll pay us back," he says in typical big-brother fashion. "And then some."

By morning I'm so ready to return to Landis that I join my brother and his two employees for their pre-dawn scrambled egg sandwiches. Karen loads me up with coffee and fruit for the road, and I head north in her ramshackle hatchback shortly after sunrise.

Still deeply shadowed and smudged with fog,
Maryland's winter browns, grays, and muted blues strike
me as the most beautiful scenery I've seen in ages. But then
my world view was bound to be sunny. Ron and I haven't
gotten along this well since...maybe ever. In a sense I
realize Corinne has had a hand in that, too, so it is with a
tempering dose of melancholy that I turn onto Route 476
and complete my northwesterly drive out to Landis.

Arriving at the AIA parking lot just before eight, I
choose an anonymous slot at the end of a center row, stash
my belongings under cover, and lock Karen's dusty brown
hatchback tight. With Ron's warnings echoing in my ears I
scrutinize my surroundings then dash into the building.

My first chore is to send the images of Jimmy Tanner
and the faked Eberly robbery to Scarp Poletta. The thirty-
second motion shots are too herky-jerky to show the
suspects faces very well—the still shots will work for
that—but at least the mpegs will prove that the boxes are
being loaded into the truck rather than removed. If my
theory proves out, I figure Scarp will owe me a steak
dinner–unless some smart-ass attorney claims the digital
shots have been computer altered.

Damn. That's exactly what an attorney will say.

Okay, okay. Not the end of the world. They still have
me as an eyewitness.

Although...

Cops, even former cops, used to be right up there with
the clergy when it came to trusted testimony, but we've had
some notable exceptions recently so even an exemplary
resume might not be enough. Especially since the
defendant might try to undermine the key witness's
credibility. Maybe have her accused of murder, something
nasty like that. Or convince her boss she's unscrupulous

and get her fired. I've seen similar scenarios play out in court, and believe me—they work.

I'm not happy to admit it, but as an explanation for what's been going on, discrediting me as a witness makes sense. It doesn't cover all the bases, but some of the other dirty tricks may have been scare tactics or power plays. I can easily imagine Jimmy Tanner's uncle, the "alleged" thief, messing with my life just to warn me away.

Which reminds me that I asked Garry to check the guy out.

My old co-worker answers as if he has Caller ID and he's been staring at the phone.

"Lauren, what have your gotten yourself into?" he asks right off the bat.

"Nothing," I fib. "Just doing my job."

"Well, if your job involves Bill Eberly, not Tanner by the way, you better watch your back. Uncle Bill is connected."

Gulp.

"Big-time connected or small potatoes connected?"

"He's not on the Most Wanted list, if that's what you mean. But if he's coming after you, does it really matter?"

I grudgingly admit he has a point, which I would have told him if he hadn't rung off to take another call.

Okay, so Uncle Bill is a bad ass, but a woman canceled my phone and ripped off my bank account. I ponder that information for a few minutes, until my brain balks.

Only thing to do when that happens is whatever feels like it should be next.

Nothing jumps out, so it's back to pounding the pavement, metaphorically speaking.

Borrowing the company phone once again, I dial up one of the three credit-rating companies and request a supervisor.

Just before hell freezes over, a Ms. Haverston tells me a weary, "Good morning." Tough job, handling complaints. To soften her up, I tell a half-truth. I say I think I've been the victim of identity theft.

After a lengthy third-degree to prove I'm me, I finally get to ask a question. "Can you please tell me exactly what put my credit on the skids?"

A bit of typing then a pause. "It appears that you have an unpaid debt dating back three years."

A little shock runs down the nerves in my back. "Really? *An* unpaid debt. Does that mean there's only one?"

"Yes."

"With whom?" I press.

"Soames Memorial Hospital."

An adrenaline surge covers me with a sudden sweat. When I was sick, my father handled all the bills; I never knew anything about what got paid and what didn't. Yet there is no getting around the obvious—my illness was the reason he began to sell off Ron's legacy—and mine—something he never would have done if money hadn't been very, very tight.

In other words, it wasn't impossible that the proceeds from the farm weren't enough. Nor was it impossible that one outstanding item slipped through the cracks.

"Can you be more specific, please?" I ask.

"It's a pharmacy invoice," the woman informs me. "Seventeen thousand seven hundred fifty seven dollars and ninety-two cents."

"Seventeen *thousand?*"

"Yes."

"Why haven't I heard anything about this before?"

The woman's silence reminds me that her company only handles information pertinent to my credit rating—if and when I've paid, that sort of thing. Still, the question make me wonder. Would my father deliberately shelter me from something like this?

Unfortunately, the answer is maybe, but that's a question for another phone call. First I need to get whatever I can out of this Haverston person.

"Can you at least tell me when your organization learned about this unpaid amount?"

An impatient sigh. "The entry was made about two weeks ago, November sixth."

"But you said the invoice dates back *three years*."

"It's a past-due statement. A summary. I can't say specifically when the expenses were incurred."

I take a breath and try to think. "All right. Then tell me this. Is it normal for your organization to get a report three years after the fact?"

The woman gives that a half-second's thought. "It does happen."

"I don't understand how..."

"An accounting oversight."

"For three years?" I'm thinking about year-end statements, audits, inventories. You don't just gloss over a seven-thousand-dollar discrepancy.

An even longer pause. "That does seem unusual."

"So tell me if I've got this right. Based on a report that's three years late, you'll totally reverse my credit rating?"

"Well, yes. If you have an unpaid debt of that size, of course."

"And has it occurred to you that if the report is incorrect or false that it would constitute fraud?"

"Not on our part, it wouldn't."

I stifle a couple of four-letter words and draw in a new breath. "Okay, supposing I can prove that the report is false, will you reinstate my credit?"

"I guess we would have to see proof. But then, yes, I suppose we would. Is that what you think happened?"

I have no idea one way or the other whether that's the case, but the timing makes my skin itch.

"Yes," I tell her, and why not? She asked for my opinion, and opinions can go either way.

"Then do you want me to mark the amount as being in dispute?"

"You can do that?"

"Isn't that why you called?"

No, but I've learned not to argue with angels. "Yes, it is," I tell her. "Thank you."

On my way to speak to David, I pass by Mike Thomas's cubicle. The car-theft specialist is on the phone, but he catches my eye and motions me over.

Hanging up, he swivels around to grunt in my face. "Do you have any idea what you've asked me to do?"

"What do you mean?" Even though I'm standing, our heads are nearly level.

"You wanted to know why Bob Battersby hates you. Don't tell me you forgot."

"No, of course not. What have you found out?"

"Not so quick. I want you to suffer first."

I fold my arms. "Oh?"

"That man has a shitload of neuroses, and you," he points a fat finger at my face, "you made me get friendly with him."

"Sorry."

"I want your firstborn named after me and the deed to your ranch. You also need to put me in your will."

"Done, done, and done. What did you find out?"

"That he blows his nose on napkins."

"Uck. Wait a minute. You had lunch with him?"

"More than once."

"I don't have all day, Mike."

"Bottom line? He invited me to The Hot Spot after work," a notorious bar in Landis's block-long "strip."

"To pick up hookers?"

"What else?"

"Why?"

"Because his mother messed up his head, that's why."

My eyes widen. "You asked him about his mother?"

"What do you think the second lunch was for? I figured a guy screwed up enough to hate beautiful women on sight—had to be about his mother."

"Wow. What'd she do?"

"Don't know—Battersby just up and left."

"So I guess The Hot Spot is out?"

The left corner of Mike's mouth rises into a rakish grin. "Who needs him?"

I know he isn't serious, so I shake my head and smile. "Thanks, man. I owe you one."

"Just tell me it helped."

I assure him it has, but in truth I'm not sure. A man who can't talk about his mother can be anything from a harmless introvert to a serial killer.

He can also be an otherwise normal male chauvinist pig.

When I tap on my boss's doorjamb, I catch him staring at his Monet water-lily mug full of sharpened pencils. The eyes he turns toward me appear blank, as if he's had a taxing weekend and isn't at all ready to concentrate on work.

I can't afford to be merciful; I tell him about the four slashed tires on the Taurus.

David's eyes steadily widen, revealing a webbing of red lines. "That's awful," he exclaims. "Were you parked in a bad neighborhood?"

"Colmar," a notoriously boring suburb.

That shocks David even more, which make me wonder how he would react to the whole story.

"So what do I do about the tires?"

"We have an arrangement with a repair shop. Write down where you left the car, and I'll call them. Do you have transportation in the meantime?"

"I borrowed something."

"Good. Very good."

Wincing as he kneads the back of his neck, he reaches for the phone.

Since I want to pay the billing department at Soames Memorial a visit, as soon as I can manage it I slip out the door.

Leaving Karen's hatchback in the hospital lot, I check my surroundings again before hurrying inside.

"No, we have nothing on the books for Lauren Beck," the female billing clerk assures me.

That's good news, of course; but it will still be a slow, irksome chore to repair my credit. The damage to my psyche is something else again.

Not so very many good checkups ago, I walked out of my doctor's office and found my way to a park bench. Sitting there eating an apple, I finally allowed myself to imagine a future without the cancer cloud over my head. It was an amazing breakthrough, like seeing the sun after forty rain-filled days and nights. I wasn't trying to delude myself; I knew deciding not to worry was only a choice, but the relief was so great I never wanted to look back.

Then along came Corinne's relapse. Mostly I was frightened for her and with her and about her, but every once in a while...

I dusted off the old arguments—Hodgkins disease was different, no reason to think her luck would be mine; only fools obsess about things that might never happen—but it was like telling myself not to think of pink elephants.

Now there is this.

An overdue drug invoice sounds so plausible—is so plausible—that I have difficulty disbelieving it. The old ghosts rise up again and circle close. So close that I have to ask the billing clerk to put her good news in writing.

"A printout? Sure." She pokes a couple of computer keys, and half a minute later I'm in possession of a statement that reads, "Amount due...zero."

Still trying to shake a sense of doom, I thank her and return to the hospital lobby. Norman Schmidt's half-joking, "Think it was something you said?" has been haunting me for a week. Also, my visit to the oncology department during Corinne's last hours rankles, not because I offended the in-house pharmacist--although I am sorry about that--but because I never got to ask all my questions. I figure Amy Dion may be more accommodating.

I find her organizing patients' charts in an area adjoining the chemotherapy waiting room.

"Lauren!" the blue-eyed brunette greets me with energy as well as surprise. "What brings you here?"

"You heard about Corinne."

"Of course. I'm so sorry. Is that what this is about?"

"Yes and no. Is there anywhere we can speak privately for a minute?" All around us it's business as usual.

She waves her head with regret. "Not right now I'm afraid."

"Do you ever get a break?"

"In my dreams."

"Let me buy you lunch?"

She tilts her head and thrusts a hip. "You've really got me curious."

"The cafeteria downstairs?"

"Sure. Twelve thirty."

With an hour and a half to kill before my lunch date, I decide to arrange a chat with the firebug/travel agent's almost ex-wife. She and her three children live in the older core section of Landis, which means the neighborhood will probably be dated and depressing, but no matter. It's close-by.

Nice surprise. Except for the trash cans along the curb, the street looks pretty good—more trees than I remember, and a nice new chain-link fence separates Dyan Shoemacher's brick and siding corner single from a strip of tidy row houses.

Yes?" she says peeking out at the stoop.

"Lauren Beck. I just called?"

Dyan grudgingly waves me in, and we settle into sturdy, blonde-armed chairs.

Three rooms deep, the house is furnished but not really decorated, so probably it's a rental. Also, the carpet looks like the stuff from my college apartment. Smells just as musty, too.

The silence, apparently, will last until I break it. "Mrs. Shoemacher..."

"I prefer Ms. Hunt."

So the divorce proceedings are coming along just fine. I've read the separation notice in the newspaper archives, the "I am no longer responsible for debts incurred by..." formality, but that doesn't always mean it's over.

"Okay then."

She has three ways to go, and the direction she chooses depends on which side of the bread got the butter. If hubby is innocent of torching his business and she thinks helping him get the insurance money will benefit her, she might embroider what little she knows. Door Number Two—the same except hubby is guilty as the day is long. Door Number Three, the unembellished truth.

"Do you happen to remember the night of November ninth?" I ask. The tape recorder is in my purse, but I'm waiting for the good stuff before bringing it out.

"Yes."

"Can you remember where you were?"

Dyan draws back and stiffens her shoulders. "What is this?"

I wave my hand. "Relax. Please. I'm just trying to establish whether you remember that night."

She eases forward in her chair, and I repeat the question.

"I was here with the kids," she says. "Where else would I be on a school night?"

"How about your husband, do you know where he was?"

"We're separated. That's the point of a separation. I don't want to know where he is."

"Okay, maybe we need to come at this from a different direction."

Suddenly my borrowed cell phone starts playing some ridiculous melody. Dilemma. The caller may be one of my sister-in-law's friends trying to reach her, or it may be one of the two people I gave the number in the last twenty-four hours.

"Excuse me," I tell my interviewee. "I have to get this."

I stand, at the same time motioning for Dyan to relax. "Hello?"

It's Scarp. Oblivious to where I am and what I'm doing, he wants details about the phony Eberly robbery, and he wants them now. "Lauren, you sweetheart. How'd you get those shots—voodoo?"

Responding to his enthusiasm, I grin like a fool while I explain about staking out the cervical strain and sprain, "the kid dumping trash in the video. I just realized what I had yesterday. Is it enough for an arrest?"

"Damn straight. The clothes dryer Eberly was loading into the truck had model numbers as big as your hand. Four of them on Eberly's inventory and four reported stolen. When the driver hears what we have, I think he'll sing like a canary. You did good, Lauren. Really heads up stuff."

"Thanks."

"One thing. The lead in this could use a written statement. Any chance we could meet at the Kynlyn Street station around four this afternoon?"

"You'll be there?"

"Sure, to introduce you. Least I can do."

Since the gesture is both out of his way and unnecessary, it seems that he wants to see me again. A little spot in my gut warms to the idea.

"See you there," he promises.

Yes, he will.

I shut the phone and try to douse my smile before returning to my conversation with Dyan Shoemacher.

"Sorry about that," I apologize. "Police business." No other way to explain the word "arrest."

One look at the pale, chastened face of the travel agent's almost-ex tells me that very word turned her around. Door Number One and Two are history. Unabridged honesty—the only way to go.

I extract the miniature recorder from my purse and set it on the end table between us. "What do you know about the fire at the Getaway Travel Agency, Ms. Hunt?"

"It's Mrs. Shoemacher, technically, at least for a little while longer," she admits, aiming her voice toward the microphone. "And I know plenty."

Of late Jerry "Getaway" Shoemacher had been increasingly despondent about his business and the effect its impending failure was having on his marriage. After losing a large and formerly loyal corporate customer, he decided that an insurance payout was the only way to save what little he had left in the world. It was a terrible risk, but he was desperate.

Jerry knew enough to light the match personally—why involve anybody else?—but his first try, using an oil-soaked paper towel, failed to ignite the flameproof drapes in his office. He had much better success with a long fuse leading into the storage closet. He just shouldn't have told Dyan he did it for her and the kids.

"Will he go to jail?" she asks me now.

You think? I want to say sarcastically, but instead I tell her it's up to law enforcement and the legal system. "My job is just the insurance piece."

Tears slip down the woman's mottled cheeks. "He's not a bad man," she recites mostly for her own benefit. "He just makes mistakes. Lots...lots of mistakes."

I don't respond. My personal opinion of a man willing to risk the lives of innocent bystanders—like Nan, the neighbor who phoned in the fire—is my personal opinion and nothing to be shared with the mother of his children. Nice people screw up all the time. They just shouldn't be surprised when they have to pay the price.

At the door I shake Dyan Shoemacher's hand and wish her luck. Time to get back to Soames for my lunch date.

Chapter 22

When Amy Dion and I queue up at the hospital cafeteria's salad bar, I build a pile of greens and douse it with balsamic vinaigrette. As an afterthought, I grab a lemon yogurt.

"Now," the oncology nurse remarks as soon as we settle into a booth. "What's this all about?"

I fold my hands at the edge of the table and look her in the eye.

"Remember when I was making a scene that day, going on about Corinne not getting the correct dosage of chemo?"

Amy dismisses that with her fork. "Please don't apologize. Lots of people..."

I flick open my hands. "Not why I'm here. I need to know if there's any chance that it's true."

Shock makes the young woman blush.

"Wild accusation, right?" I concede, "but please humor me for a minute. What if it *were* true?"

The nurse lowers her fork and glances away. When she looks back again, her eyes are filled with pity. "Lauren," she begins, "I know you loved Corinne, but..."

"No. No, please listen. A woman was working at the pharmacy window right beside us. Remember? She was eavesdropping so bad we had to move?"

"Sara, our pharmacist," Amy acknowledges. "Everybody's nosy around here, Lauren. It comes with the territory."

I shake my head to disagree. "This time may be different."

"Why?"

"Because someone's been harassing me ever since— systematically shutting down my life." I explain about my cell phone, my checking account, my credit. I tell her I live in Corinne's attic and that I can't go home, "because somebody convinced Corinne's daughter that I had something to do with her mother's death."

"That's absurd"

"Tell that to the police."

"The police! You can't be serious."

My silence tells her I am.

"Oh, hell," the nurse laments. "Even if they asked me, it wouldn't help you. I wasn't there."

"But you believe me?"

She considers that. "My instincts say yes. My head says if you did anything to Corinne—and I'm not saying you did—it would have been because you loved her."

We're picking our way across rocky territory here, so I spend some time eating, time that allows Amy to finish making up her mind about me.

"You've had a rough couple of weeks," she remarks a moment later.

I roll my eyes and sigh, more relieved than I care to admit that she landed on my side of the fence. "I'll get over losing Corinne...eventually. But the other things...I hate feeling so...so disconnected, unplugged. None of my tools work anymore—I don't *have* any tools. I don't even have a home."

"Almost sounds like a rape," the nurse observes, which tells me she hasn't spent all of her career caring for cancer patients.

"Yes and no," I demur. "My ego's still functioning...after a fashion."

"I only said it sounded like a rape. I didn't say he succeeded."

"He."

"I can't imagine a woman trying to ruin a person like that, can you?"

"Yes, I'm afraid I can."

Amy sneaks a glance at the cafeteria clock. "Tell me more about why you're here."

I push my food aside. "The other day," I say, "I came because I believed something was wrong with Corinne's treatment. But then, like you, I realized how preposterous that sounded. Who could be that...that monstrous? Inconceivable, right? But some people are monsters, Amy. Honest to God. Some of them really are."

"For money."

"Usually for money," I agree. Jerry Schumacher and his pile of cinders, for instance.

She watches me a long moment then looks away. "It's still pretty hard to swallow."

Another long moment and then her chin lifts, her shoulders draw back. "I administer those drugs myself," she says with a shudder. "If something was the matter with them...the ramifications would be...it could ruin the hospital."

"I know. I've been thinking the same thing. Believe me. Plus there are other, much more likely, explanations for what's been happening."

Without naming names I give her the rundown on Bob Battersby, Jimmy Tanner, and the Eberly robbery photos. It amazes me how few answers I have.

"The only way I know to get out from under all of this is to operate the way I did when I was a cop—examine every possibility, no matter how remote, until I come across the one piece of the puzzle that puts everything else in focus."

"Medicine's like that, too."

My eyebrows rise, and Amy laughs. So of course I do, too. Then we settle into comfortable smiles.

"How can I help?" she asks.

"Talk to me. Forget about how improbable it sounds. Tell me how it could be done."

"Water down the doses?" She does a quick surveillance of the room. "It would be easy," she admits with a grimace.

"How easy?"

She crumbles her napkin. "We pretty much get what we need off the shelf, so the dilution would have to be done at the source—the outside pharmacy that makes up the IV bags." She gives a little shrug. "Really any sick bastard pharmacist could do it."

I ask which pharmacy supplies Soames Memorial.

"East Side. We've had a contract with them for about five years."

"Okay. How can we find out whether anybody's been tampering with the drugs they send to Soames?"

"I'll talk to our Cancer Registrar, Kathy Parker. Her whole job is keeping track of our cancer statistics. If I tell her it's for one of the doctors, she can give me a printout."

I wave my head. "Better not involve anybody we don't have to." I caution.

"You mean the doctor? Why not?"

"Because if something nasty is going on, whoever is behind it could become very dangerous very fast."

Amy's lips press into a stubborn line. "If it is true, then patients are dying."

Behind that sentence I hear the influence of the Hippocratic oath, and it makes me want to retract everything I've said. As persuasively as possible, I remind Amy that the chemo remark was only one of many things I've done that could have triggered the harassment—witnessing a crime, thwarting some less-than-honest customers, upstaging my co-workers—being more of a daughter to Corinne than her daughter.

Yet even as I make my case, I hear myself saying *very dangerous very fast.* So far, the perp's only scare has come from me, a woman too distraught to be taken seriously. Insuring that I won't become an even greater threat is a no-brainer, especially if big bucks are at stake. On the other hand, Amy's inquiries won't be construed as harmless or even accidental, and if anything happens to her I'll never forgive myself.

"On second thought, this is probably just a waste of time," I recant. "Maybe we should forget the whole thing."

"No!" she objects. "I want to look into this. I need to...for myself."

"It's just a theory, Amy. And a pretty wild one at that."

"Maybe," an attempt to humor me, because her resolve doesn't budge. "But...I've had this feeling for a while now." She pinches her fingers together. "I came this close to asking the other nurses about it, then I decided it was probably just me being me. But now..."

"What feeling, Amy?"

"That we're losing more than we're winning." She sighs heavily and contemplates her hands. "Still, I'm an oncology nurse, you know? Part of my job is not giving in to negativity."

She checks the clock again. "Yikes! I've gotta go. How can I reach you?"

I write Karen's cell phone number on a napkin; Amy gives me her home number on another. We dump our lunch refuse and leave our trays on the adjacent stack. Then I walk with her as far as the elevators.

"Sara," she says. "Another reason I hope Richard is innocent," she remarks.

"Who's Richard?"

"Richard Kiel, owner of East Side."

"Sara and he are friends?"

"She thinks so," the nurse confides with a crooked grin. "He butters her up with candy and movie tickets, stuff like that. I think he's just trying to keep his contract, but Sara thinks he's interested, you know? So on top of everything else, I hope it's nothing—for her sake."

"Me, too."

We say our good-byes as Amy steps into an elevator. My head is buzzing, but somehow I cross the lobby and exit through the sliding glass doors.

Richard Kiel.

Who is the owner of the East Side pharmacy?

Richard Kiel.

And who is the only person who will profit by diluting the chemotherapy drugs?

Richard Kiel, the owner of the East Side pharmacy.

Guess where I'm going next.

First off, the East Side pharmacy is not a retail store. It is a narrow storefront operation sandwiched between a second-hand music outlet and a hairdresser on the brief business section of the main street of Dean, Pennsylvania. Originally the size of a suburban village, Dean has exceeded its boundaries the same way a toddler outgrows its crib. As a result, who-knows-who rents who-knows-what if it happens to be a useful size and the price is right.

Parking anywhere near the center of town is a creative challenge only minimally addressed by two public lots five blocks apart. I leave Karen's hatchback in the nearest one, perhaps a hundred yards from the pharmacy on the same side of the street. Just in case Richard Kiel knows what I look like, I zip my windbreaker up to the throat and wrap a scarf over my head. Then I begin to stroll back and forth along the block, pretending to be window-shopping. Glancing through plate-glass windows left over from the East Side's former life gives me a pretty good idea of what's going on inside.

Shelves run along both walls and down the middle of the room, and three women and one man move about retrieving what they need. The pharmacists or assistants, for no one person appears to be in charge, each have a work station where they complete orders and attended to recordkeeping. On my second go-by I notice an open doorway to a rear room that probably contains more of the same. In other words, the place looks like any other busy pharmacy minus the customers and cashier.

To avoid suspicion, I cross the street. A movie theater directly opposite Kiel's establishment has nothing playing early on a Monday afternoon; but its entrance is out of the wind, so I pace back and forth there, checking my watch and trying to look as if I'm waiting for someone.

Coming up on three o'clock I notice an older man standing in the front window of the pharmacy. A couple minutes later he's joined by a second also older man, who entered from the street. The first is of the tall, spry variety, the second lumbers like an old overweight dog. They have to be deliverymen newly arrived for work.

Yep, deliverymen. A sudden flurry of activity—boxes of bags being handed out, assignments given. I decide to follow the slow old dog, maybe try to get a word with him a safe distance away from East Side. If I'm lucky, I'll get what I need to convince Amy to drop her inquiries. If not...well, I don't want to think about if not.

The door opens and out comes Isaac, my nickname for the tall, spry retiree. I squint hard, but I can no longer see my preferred "old dog" through the window.

No choice but to go with the tail I drew. Paralleling Isaac and his box of prescriptions, I stay even with him until he enters a side alley. When he stops at the second parked car, an aging black Ford Crown Victoria, I sprint for the hatchback, all the while thanking the municipal gods for choosing parking meters over attendants. I'm able to fire up my car and screech around to face Main, hopefully while Isaac is still unlocking his boat, stowing the box of prescriptions, and mentally mapping out his route.

The Crown Victoria cruises past my nose before I can blink.

Traffic. I need to go left, but a parade of after-school moms get in my way.

Turning at last, I join the crowd jammed up by a traffic light at Bethlehem Pike—just in time to watch the Crown Vic ooze around the corner and pick up speed. Nearly biting my tongue with frustration, I finally get my turn; but three others have preceded me. Three chances to get left behind.

For a quarter mile Bethlehem Pike arches toward the right. Residential side streets feed off it, and I decide to gamble on cutting through them. Quick right. Hard left. Kids may be out with bikes or balls. Dogs. Baby carriages. But this is November and the temptation to be outdoors isn't great. I floor it where I can and back off drastically when I can't.

I make it back to the pike just in time to see the third car off the Crown Vic pass by. I've gained nothing and almost lost completely. There has to be another way.

Two miles later I figure out where Isaac is going—to a big retirement home five miles ahead. Perfect potential customer for East Side. I relax enough to tell myself it isn't the end of the world if I guessed wrong, tomorrow is another day, and all that. Meanwhile, I keep tabs on Isaac as best I can.

He makes no unexpected moves. Two of the cars between us turn off, giving me a cushion of one tall blue van. This, too, finally signals for a driveway, and the rest is smooth sailing.

"Sunrise Hill Nursing Home" is spelled out in metallic letters mounted on brick at the bottom of a rolling lawn. Sidewalks perfect for wheelchairs ring the driveway. Convenient parking for visitors. I stick Karen's hatchback in the first available slot and run for the doorway where Isaac has stopped his big black sedan. He's still preoccupied by the prescription bags when I catch up, so I use the few seconds' leeway to enter the lobby through the automatic doors. Now I'll appear to be leaving as he comes in.

We meet face to face on the sidewalk.

"Hey!" I call out in a friendly fashion. "Don't you work for Richard Kiel?"

Isaac is perhaps six-foot four and maybe twenty-inches wide. What long straight hair he has is gunmetal gray, and his sunken cheeks need a shave.

"Wha?" he responds, showing me some imperfect teeth.

"Richard Kiel. East Side Pharmacy. You work for them right?"

"Uh, yeah?"

"Wow, that boss of yours is one hard guy to pin down. I've been trying to invite him to dinner for weeks. Is he away or something?" As I speak, I dance back and forth to prevent the man's escape.

"Lady, you got the wrong guy," the deliveryman tells me with a peeved tone. "Richard's old enough to be your father."

"So? My husband and I can't invite him and his wife to dinner?"

The deliveryman's already narrow face narrows some more. "I'm telling you, you got the wrong guy. The boss is divorced."

"Oh, no! What a shame, she was so…so nice."

"Lady, I gotta get back to work."

"Just a second. You are from East Side, right?" He can scarcely deny it since the pharmacy name is printed all over the bags he's holding. "And Richard is the owner. So can you tell me whether he's been at work much lately, because…"

"He's been in and out," the man allows, bobbing left and right in an effort to break free. "Took a couple of half days, that's all. Now if you'll excuse me."

I step aside.

Do I like what I'd just learned? I saunter back to the hatchback and think about it. Free time for the potential perp to screw around with me falls into the category of "opportunity," an essential ingredient for proving guilt. Yet the pharmacist may be using his off time for any number of innocent activities. I'm conflicted about this whole line of inquiry, torn about calling Amy off.

She catches me on Karen's cell phone while I'm driving back to the office.

"Just wanted you to know," she says as I curb the car to listen. "Kathy, our cancer registrar, gave me a disc and a printout of some patient information. A to C, just a start, but here's the thing. She really doesn't buy your theory,

Lauren. She's been here for two years and she hasn't noticed one single problem."

"Was she miffed?" I ask, responding to the strain in the nurse's voice.

"Yeah, a little. I blamed it on you. I hope you don't mind."

"Quite all right. I'm totally nuts, in case you hadn't noticed."

Amy laughs, but our business is too sobering and she quickly falls silent.

"Still, it won't hurt to double check," I suggest. She already has the information, so why not read it?

"Oh, I will," and in that short phrase I hear echoes of the idealist who is concerned about Soames's cancer mortality rate.

"Do me one more favor?" I push, returning to my own agenda. "Label the disc 'Christmas card list' or something like that, will you?"

"You're really creeping me out here."

"Sorry. I'm just naturally suspicious. But please do be careful, Amy. I already regret involving you in this."

"No problem. Like Kathy said, it's probably nothing. Anyway, you want to meet at my place tonight? I can show you the stuff."

"Sounds good," I say, shoving my qualms aside.

She gives me directions to her apartment then at the last minute invites me to stay over. "You said you can't go back to Corinne's," she reminds me, "and I've been wondering what you've been doing."

"Sleeping on floors," I answer, to save a long explanation. "Thanks."

Then I remember the Eberly deposition. "Does it matter when I get there?"

"Not really. I never know when I'll finish up either. Key's behind the base of the front-door light fixture," she informs me. "Just tilt it up and it'll fall out. Make yourself at home."

An ally, I think as I shut my phone.

That's good, right?

Chapter 23

Curiosity is driving me nuts, so I stop by the office to run a computer check on Richard Kiel before my meeting at the Kynlyn Street police station. During mid afternoon nobody much is around. I kick my purse under the desk and keep my jacket on.

On the surface, the pharmacist is quite a contrast to Jimmy Tanner's Uncle Bill. No rented Mercedes for this guy—Kiel drives a year-old purchased Cadillac and belongs to two country clubs. Although he and his wife divorced about a year ago, somehow he's managed to retain his primary residence, a handful of investment properties, and a forty-five-foot sailboat. Makes me suspect that the missus was unfaithful and Richard's lawyer made hay of it. Or the more charitable explanation—his kids are grown and the ex promptly remarried.

Unfortunately, nothing on the screen tells me whether Richard Kiel came by his comforts legitimately or at the expense of a long list of terminal cancer patients.

Nothing says he's been using his half-days off to shipwreck my life either.

Still, I'm disappointed. I'm weary of wild goose chases; I want results.

I know, I know. One part inspiration, six parts perspiration. Just stick with the basics, Lauren, and keep your eyes and ears open.

In the meantime, my meeting with Scarp.

The Kynlyn Street police station is a gray stone relic that says early nineteen hundreds to me. I park in a visitors slot and trot toward the sidewalk. Two large clumps of dried out decorative grass rattle like chain mail as I pass; and high above an American flag flaps in the afternoon's steady breeze.

Inside, the hodgepodge supports my guesstimate of the building's age. Floors of the original hardwood worn into pale traffic patterns guide you between and around sectioned-off work stations. Windows are the antiquated casement variety with bars very obviously added later. On each desk are wire in-baskets beside the computer terminals, and the fragrances of coffee and old dust hang in the air. I haven't been back here in years.

A female dispatcher/receptionist directs me to the opened door of a conference room, which is empty but for an oblong table surrounded by institutional metal chairs and the two men waiting for me. I slow my pace to a ladylike walk, halting just short of the end of the table.

Breaking off his conversation, Poletta turns my way, lifts the left corner of his intriguing mouth and says, "Hey, Lauren. Thanks for coming." He has on softened light blue jeans over black motorcycle boots, a black mock-turtleneck and a richly textured black and brown tweed sport coat. Some pale blue flecks in the jacket's fabric make the whole bit work so well I would have enjoyed a snapshot for my bedroom wall. Better yet, an oversized poster.

I nod hello.

"Hey, come in. Come in," urges the municipal detective named Clarence Weisman.

"He caught the Eberly burglary case," Scarp adds to complete the introduction.

Weisman is about my size, which is to say slightly tall for a woman but small for a man. He has on a white oxford button-down under a misshapen navy blazer that probably does duty year-round. By far his most arresting feature is a pair of ripe-olive eyes, which he blinks at me in welcome. "You really saved our asses here, Lauren. May I call you Lauren?"

"Certainly, and you're welcome. It was really just a piece of good luck."

"Unbelievable luck." Weisman snorts and then laughs, showing me that's exactly what he thinks it was. "Julie will be here in a second to record your statement. Get anybody coffee while we're waiting?"

Both of us accept, and Weisman swaggers out of the room.

Scarp catches me looking skeptical. "He's really sweet when you get to know him."

"Do I have to?"

Poster-boy sniffs at that and shifts his shoulders slightly left and right, just realigning himself to talk to me, but the roll of his muscles makes my mind go blank.

"Dinner after this?" he suggests.

"Probably," I reply.

"No," he says. "You and me. You want to have dinner together?"

I look at his face then, and my lips part. Naturally, that's the moment a woman who weighs two hundred and bench presses at least that chooses to walk in. Her business garb is an unlikely mustard hue and she carries a steno machine that resembles the ones they use in court.

"Sorry I'm late," she huffs. "Traffic on 202."

"Yes," I say, and Scarp mumbles something that sounds like "Umph?"

"Yes, afterward," I turn and tell him unequivocally, and he lifts the left corner of his mouth again and readjusts his shoulders.

Weisman returns and distributes coffees in cardboard cups. Mine tastes like scorched shoe leather, but it keeps my throat working long enough to respond to the questions. "What were you doing in the parking lot of the Meadow Woods Shopping Center? How long were you surveilling your subject before you noticed the truck behind Eberly Electronics? What prompted you to take the photographs you subsequently sent to Detective Poletta? To your knowledge did anyone alter or enhance the photographs in any way?" All of that and more. I sip sludge and answer succinctly and try to keep my mind off temptation.

Eventually Clarence stands and looks down his nose at me. "Thanks for your time, Lauren. Seriously, you saved our asses."

In my experience nobody says "seriously" like that unless they're lying, so I tell him "My pleasure" in kind. Then for the hell of it I make him shake my hand in a sissy-prissy manner before departing with Scarp by my side.

As soon as we're safely outdoors, my dinner-date asks if I always mock my superiors like that, "or were you just having fun now that you're not on the force?"

"Why Rhett, how you do go on."

Scarp snorts and steers me between the clumps of dead grass. Twilight has come and gone, and the halogen overheads make everything look fake. When we reach the side of my car, Scarp opens the door and inquires if the Valley Forge Brewing Company is okay for dinner.

I know first-hand what public servants get paid, so I tell him that will be great.

"I'll follow you."

"I'll go slow," he says in a bedroom voice. At least it sounds like a bedroom voice to me.

"Promise?" I beg, and he snorts again.

One of the many microbreweries that recently sprang from the Philadelphia soil, the Valley Forge Brewing Company purveys its product from a typical strip-mall restaurant. To distinguish itself, it has a shiny beer brewing apparatus behind glass in the entranceway and two steps up to the restaurant floor. For ambience they've lowered the lights.

Better and better, a waitperson named George seats us well back in the middle of the room where we are surrounded by the same quantity of children as Peter Pan. I order the Yankee pot pie and a beer margarita to start.

"I thought you only drank beer," Scarp remarks after the waiter departs.

"Red wine usually." We've begun to lean across the table toward each other, a feeble attempt to create privacy where none exists.

"But weren't you drinking beer at Casey's last week?"

How sweet, noticing date-like details way back then. "I was pretending to be one of the guys."

"Oh? And how does that work for you, being one of the guys?"

I wriggle in a little closer. "You tell me."

The homicide detective waves his big dark head and frowns. "Not well at all, I shouldn't think."

My smile goes a little lopsided. "Now that you mention it, the beer trick went over better when I was armed."

Scarp spreads his hands in a see-that gesture. "And you women say we're terrible at picking up signals."

Smiles all around when the waiter brings our drinks, but then I decide to clear away a potential stumbling block. I inquire whether I'm still a murder suspect.

Scarp inhales then drinks deeply from his beer before replying. "Yeah, sort of."

"Is this," I gesture around me, "compromising your investigation?"

The homicide detective looks me frankly in the eye. "Close examination of the subject? Not at all. Anyhow, I've got another reason for meeting with you...one on one, so to speak."

"Oh?"

"Yeah. It's a safety issue. Information you need to have."

"Oh?"

"Yeah. About your electronics guy, Eberly. You want it now or later?"

"Now, please."

Scarp sighs and starts playing with this paper coaster, running it around and around between his fingers. Then abruptly he tosses it aside and blurts, "Eberly did some juvenile time with Morris Squillante."

I blink and tilted my head. "You'll have to bring me up to speed."

"Sure. Here's the thing. Squillante runs a tri-state auto theft ring—we're close to nailing him, but we're not ready yet. You know how that goes."

"Yes."

"Squillante has friends with gambling interests, also a few girls down in the city." That would be prostitutes.

"Go on."

"We think Eberly is pretty straight, just one drunk-and-disorderly since juvie, one minor assault—clocked some guy in a bar. Stupid stuff. But we've seen him with Squillante off and on for years, and now because of the store heist we learned that he's in debt to Squillante's gambling guys." Scarp actually laughs. "Knucklehead notion—Eberly was counting on the leg-breakers to leave him alone until after his insurance company paid up."

This is more detail than Garry gave me, which is intriguing in itself. "Interesting," I admit, "but what does it have to do with me?"

Scarp's aspect hardens so fast it's frightening. "You figure it out," he challenges. "An insurance investigator who just happens to be on the scene when the heist is going down? Helluva coincidence, don't you think?"

So it's worse than I thought. "The gambling guys think my whiplash assignment was bogus, that I was investigating Eberly as an avenue to them?"

Scarp shrugs. "Maybe. Or maybe they buy that you were there by chance. But you're still an insurance investigator who used to be a cop. What do they figure you're going to do next?"

"Screw them up."

"Exactly. And what *did* you do?"

"I screwed them up."

"Correct. Since Eberly ain't gonna earn much in prison—yes, they're screwed. And yes, the tough guys probably blame you."

"Fine. So I'm a pain in their ass, but it's over now, isn't it?"

"That depends on who Eberly really was to them— we're talking both Squillante and his buddies now. If he was more than a customer, more than just an occasional errand boy, then I don't know what they'll do about you. And that's my point. These people can't afford to show weakness. Ignoring the fact that you cost them money would play very badly in their circle. So watch your back, Lauren. Eberly isn't even behind bars yet, you hear me? That's what I wanted to tell you. Be very careful for a while."

I regard my table companion with different eyes. My ego doesn't want him to be just a nice guy who isn't above a harmless flirtation.

Which reminds me how often my ego got me in trouble back when I was actually dating.

To hell with my libido. Better a flesh wound now than a fatal one down the road.

"Why didn't Clarence tell me any of this?"

Scarp looks me in the eye again, and it's all the answer I need. Weisman wrote off my photographs as dumb luck and, as a consequence, labeled me with a mental epithet that rhymed. According to his way of thinking I'm perfectly safe so long as I don't cruise bars after dark.

The waiter has come and gone. "My food looks good," Scarp remarks. "How about yours?"

I try a bite of the Yankee pot pie, but my mind isn't paying attention.

I ask if Scarp wants to know what's happened to me since Corinne's funeral.

He gives me a nod and smile, so I relate the history of my last two weeks while we both work on our food.

Scarp looks off into the distance before presenting his summation. "You've got Nina gunning for you with or without a little help from a friend..." both of us question whether her tipster exists, "...then you've got the guy at work you irritated by breathing."

"I solved his case."

"...and made him look stupid. Then you've got the whiplash kid, Jimmy, who may or may not have asked his sort-of-connected uncle to cut you down to size."

"... and Jimmy's girlfriend, whose claim got denied, too." While I speak I'm also tying the Bob Battersby/prostitute threads together.

"Anybody else?"

His expression says he's kidding; but I'm done. I confess that I'd made a stupid remark to a Soames oncology nurse in front of a witness.

"What sort of stupid remark?"

That slander problem again.

"I questioned whether Corinne had gotten all the care she deserved."

Understandably, Scarp can't cut through that veil with a machete, so he says the only thing anybody could say. "You're probably not the first, or the last, to do that. People go a little nuts where their loved ones are concerned."

"Don't I know it." We both seem to be flashing back to Nina's outburst at the funeral and our escape into the countryside.

"You really can't stay in your apartment?" he asks. I shake my head, and he nods. "So you want to come home with me, or what?"

A guilty smile takes over my face, and my companion's grin broadens in response.

"It isn't far," he teases.

Fifteen minutes later, I ease Karen's hatchback to a stop at the curb of his townhouse and step out into the early evening air.

But then I look at the man hunting through his keys in the porch light and realize my whole body has gone cold. I'm actually shivering.

"Nope," I tell myself, and my blood starts to flow again. "No thank you. Not tonight. Maybe never." That last one was just relief talking, but I'm already in the car and driving away.

Scarp is a detective; he'll figure it out.

Chapter 24

From Scarp's front curb I proceed straight to Amy Dion's. I'll be later than she expected, but we left the time of my arrival pretty open-ended.

The apartment complex where the oncology nurse lives is H-shaped, with two center stairwells and two entrance lobbies. The goal was probably a more personal feel and more windows, but the building's configuration makes finding your destination way too hard. Plus I have real concerns about security. Something to keep in mind when I start looking for another place of my own.

Four A is up and to the back of the left-hand half of the H. A rear stairwell faces the elevator and the next closest apartment is around the corner. Although I seem to be alone, I hear nearby movement almost as soon as I step into the hall, a sort of draft on the back of my neck. Just to be safe, I finger the Glock out of my purse and slip it into my jacket pocket. I also hold my breath and listen for a minute, but the noise doesn't repeat.

Eight o'clock. Amy's probably home by now, so I give her door a polite tap.

No response, so after a moment I try again.

Nothing, so I follow my host's instructions and lift the light fixture by the door.

A key drops out just as she said it would. I retrieve it from the floor and begin to put it in the lock, but I hear that sound behind me again. It comes from somewhere in the hall, I can't see where.

I listen for another minute but soon realize that Scarp's warnings have me spooked. I've even grabbed for the Glock again. Ridiculous.

Yet when I turn the door key and push, the chain bolt is on and I hear a gasp. Something is wrong.

"Amy? It's me, Lauren," I call through the gap.

"Go away," she shouts back. "I changed my mind." She sounds physically afraid of me.

"Okay," I assure her, "but can you at least tell me why?"

"Just...just go away. Please."

Unfair rejection–it always feels the same. My heart hammers against my ribs, and I've broken out in a sweat. "What about the printouts, Amy? Did you look at them?"

"There's no fraud, Lauren. Kathy didn't find a thing, and neither did I. Now go away. Please. I don't want to have to call the police."

Rounding the corner, a woman in a green wool coat halts so fast she looks as if she smacked into a wall.

"Oh, no. Oh, no, no, no," she repeats as she backs away and then runs. I hear her receding footsteps and the slam of a distant door. If Amy hasn't already called 9-1-1, that one will.

I scowl, trying to work out the reason.

Then I notice the gun in my hand, hear the echo of Amy's final, "... *call the police.*"

My breath rushes from my lungs and my head spins. Forcing myself to focus, I return the gun to my purse. I shut Amy's door and hide her key behind the light fixture.

Then I run down the service stairs and out into the night.

Chapter 25

Not knowing if anybody saw me run to the hatchback, I drive in long slow circles like a lost old lady. It's dark. Who will know that I'm choking the steering wheel and cursing my own stupidity?

Amy Dion's been turned. At noon she was my ally; now she's scared to death of me. Big loss. *Huge* loss, but what can I do?

I have to assume the police know about the "Incident in the Hall," which they will less generously describe as "Intimidation with a fire-arm," or perhaps "Attempted..." who knows what? If they catch up with me, no way will they buy my story.

One jittery loop and then two. Any corner might conceal a roadblock, any side street harbor a black and white. When a van pulls into a service station, I make certain it stops at a pump. A shop light goes off, and I flinch.

I tell myself this is crazy, that the cops are either after me or they aren't, that nothing I do or don't do will matter much either way.

Another mile without sirens and I'm settled down enough to consider my destination. Every option has risks, so I figure I might as well go where I want to be. If what I think is going on is going on, Scarp may actually hear me out; and, let's face it—who else will?

Leaving Karen's hatchback three blocks away, I slink along the shadows to Scarp's townhouse. Then I take a deep breath and ring the bell.

Just when I'm about to bolt, he opens the door. His face shows both surprise and distrust; but on the bright side, he doesn't arrest me.

"Hey, Lauren," he says, looking me up and down. "How you doin'?" He wears a gray sweat suit complete with sweat, as if he's been working off excess testosterone lifting weights.

"Been better," I admit. "May I come in?"

Scarp shrugs and steps back into the light, revealing what I initially missed—disappointment and hurt.

I'm all set to apologize; but his arm pulls me in, and his mouth smothers mine. One touch of his tongue and I forget whatever I was about to say.

The next thing I know we're trying to undress without letting go, kissing and laughing and stumbling for the stairs. I throw my bra at his crotch and he carries me the rest of the way.

Flopped on his bed, we smile goofy smiles into each other's eyes. Then just before he turns out the light, he touches my cheek with his thumb.

"You're crying," he says. "How come?"

"Just happy," I confess, because right this minute it's true.

Thursday morning. I'm half awake. I start to roll over, bump into a warm body, and scream. Well, not scream exactly. Yelp? I make an involuntary sound loud enough to jerk Scarp from a sound sleep into a sitting position. If his gun had been on the night table, he'd have pointed it at me. But then he is a cop. When I was on the job, I'd have reacted the same way.

"Sorry," I say, referring the yelp.

"S'okay," he mutters. His throat pulses visibly, and he's rubbing his eyes. "Now I don't have to wait for the alarm."

The clock in question reads five thirty-six. I almost apologize again, but Scarp has begun to kiss my fingertips and my skin is taut all the way to the tops of my feet.

Last night was all about discovery and abandon, but this morning I'm so self-conscious I feel brittle. A credit to his patience, Scarp demolishes my inhibitions with humor and, I must confess, extraordinary skill. And, yes, the results are well worth the extra effort. The Brent W. Cahill curse is history—saying "yes" is once again an option.

I'm just not sure it will still be an option with Scarp, not after he plugs into the cop network and learns about Amy Dion's hallway.

Still, I hold out hope.

Since my hours are flexible, he showers while I start the coffee. Then, curious to see what I missed the night before, I check out the downstairs, and I like what I see.

In the narrow living room is a squared-off sofa covered in a textured deep brown; on the end table, a white ceramic lamp with a sensually curved base. Scarp seems to own only one piece of art, a blurry watercolor that resembles wild horses. The bookshelves display forensic texts and tomes on ballistics, plus a row of hard-boiled best-sellers— the stuff I used to read for laughs. It all fits with my assessment of the man–a workaholic content to wait for what he wants.

Back in the bedroom I wait while he snaps his service piece into his underarm holster before handing him his coffee.

He grunts and sets the mug aside. Shrugs into another tweed sport coat with brown flecks a little lighter than his eyes. "Where you gonna be today?"

"Just finished an arson case," I answer, choosing the most boring chore that comes to mind. "Gotta write the report." That isn't my plan, but I don't dare share my other investigation with him yet.

I follow Poletta down to his living room and watch him unchain the door.

"Be careful out there," I joke, referencing the ubiquitous *Hill Street Blues* reruns.

Scarp turns around and places two strong hands on my biceps. His dark curly hair is still wet and perfectly in place. His tanned, lived-in face is smooth from his shave, his expression just philosophical enough to reveal nothing.

"Lauren Beck," he marvels. "Who'd have thunk it?" He smiles while his eyebrows lower in honor of the irony.

"We're not exactly the odd couple."

"No?" he inquires, which reminds me. Men think they have instincts, too.

We kiss good-bye, long and soft, and I think, "Nice. This is very...very nice."

When he's gone, I stare at the door until my legs are ready to obey my brain.

In the shower I sing the only two lines I remember from Willie Nelson's *On the Road Again* until my body is squeaky clean.

As I shampoo my hair, I begin to wonder if I should go back to Amy Dion's. Maybe in the light of day she'll feel safe enough to tell me who frightened her—and what they said.

Nope. Bad idea. A good way to get thrown in jail.

She has probably left for work anyhow, which was where we'd been seen together and most likely where she was approached. "Oh, by the way, Corinne Wilder didn't die of pneumonia after all." Then the persuasive details. A staff member "saw me" doing something that supported the euthanasia theory. Or, worse, the forensic techs "discovered evidence" that points to me. It amounts to Nina's favorite fantasy, and I wonder whether she has a hospital connection I don't know about.

Regardless, manufactured proof would be tough to refute. Anybody visiting Corinne would have touched things around her, and I visited her as frequently as the rules allowed. So my concerns are real; facts are often subject to interpretation, just listen in on any trial.

Still, by the time I'm dressed I've convinced myself to let the whole Amy business cool off a bit. Scarp went out of his way to warn me about Bill Eberly's connection to Morris Squillante, so that's probably the more serious threat.

I lock the townhouse door behind me. Then I drive to work as vigilantly as if I'm back on patrol.

Chapter 26

My safe arrival at the AIA parking lot reassures me that nobody is watching for the hatchback. Me, maybe. The hatchback—no. Which is why I eyeball everything in sight and even bend down to peek under the nearby cars before I hustle inside.

Like zebras to a watering hole other employees are converging on the lobby, too. Only my twelfth day on the job and already I recognize many of them. At the elevator a few even nod and smile.

Then I get to the ninth floor hallway and come face to face with Bob Battersby. Fat face ignited with glee, he leans his stuffed blue shirt close enough to whisper, "Had any hyssie fits lately?" If another investigator hadn't been passing by, I'd have given him the finger.

David loiters in the doorway to his glass house watching his worker bees arrive. He brightens when he sees me.

"The Taurus is back," he announces, tossing me my neon-pink key ring.

"Wonderful. Where is it?"

"Northwest corner of the lot, third row in."

I thank him, and he gestures me into his visitor's chair. We talk a bit about my open cases, and he tells me he's given me four more.

"I know you've only been here two weeks," he says with a touch to his pouty lip, "but you've got to pick up the pace L.B. Chop, chop, chop or else chop, chop. Capish?"

"Absolutely." An inward groan. "I'll do my best."

An hour later the arson report is wrapped up, so I choose another case that should be easy to close. A tree limb supposedly fell and smashed a large decorative window, but for some reason the claim was flagged. I need to get myself over there to see why, but there's a problem. My company car is not where David said it would be.

With the creepy sensation that I'm being watched, I walk every aisle and check every corner of the vast employee lot, but no black Taurus with the right license number is anywhere to be seen.

I return to the ninth floor and tap on David's doorjamb. Fortunately, he's alone. "Did you actually see the Taurus after they delivered it?"

"What?" He's been reading something on his computer and hasn't completely made the transition. "See it? No. Why do you ask?"

"Because I checked the whole lot, and it isn't there."

David grabs for his phone. "We'll just call and ask." He dials as he speaks.

"Yes. David Willard at AIA. Tell me again where you put that Taurus." A couple grunts and uh-huhs. "Well, my investigator says she can't find it." An alarmed glance my way and a final, "Thanks, Mark.

"Mark says he parked it three rows from the back about five cars from the end in the northwest corner. Put it there about four-thirty yesterday afternoon. He remembers because he was hoping to beat the traffic."

"It isn't there now.".

"Let's look together."

We repeat my search with the same result. Lots of company cars, none of them mine.

"If that isn't the damnest thing," David remarks when we meet up on the sidewalk. "You want to call the police, or should I?"

"You," I tell him. "I've got work to do, remember?"

Back on our floor I gather up the printouts for my new cases and get ready to leave; but then I spy Mike Thomas perched on his oversized chair pecking at his keyboard.

"Just the person I was hoping to see."

He pretends to groan. "Who do you want me to buddy up with, this time? Ossama bin Laden?"

"Nobody. I need to learn about auto theft."

His face splits into a smile. "How long do you have?"

"Five minutes."

"You young people have no tenacity, no soul..."

"Four minutes."

Thomas rolls his blue eyes upward as if consulting a cloudy muse. "Smash and grab."

"No glass at the scene."

"Okay, then magnets to circumvent the lock pads."

"Taurus."

"Your company car?"

"Yes. David's phoning it in."

"I'll go talk to him."

"Me first..."

Mike needs no additional urging. He launches into a lecture about transponders, shaved keys, wafers, websites that sell keys, infrared systems, and losses amounting to three billion dollars a year. "Essentially, if Detroit can invent it, the punks can disable it. And will, sooner or later."

I learn about proximity cards, which look like credit cards but are electronically recognized by only one vehicle. I learn that those popular anti-theft "clubs" can be circumvented by sawing through the steering wheel. And I learn that a thief with foresight and patience might even order a replacement key from a dealership.

I thank Mike and escape with my suspicion confirmed. If somebody wanted my car, they could get it. The real question was who on earth would want it? Tauruses are nice, but they can be found all over the place, and the majority of them are in better condition than my secondhand company hack. So rule out a random snatch for parts. This is another round of Get Lauren Beck.

Auto theft, I recite to myself as I make my way out to the hatchback. Auto theft. Where else has that been mentioned recently?

At dinner when Scarp informed me that Bill Eberly is friendly with Morris Squillante, who just happens to run a tri-state auto-theft ring. A word from Jimmy Tanner to Uncle Bill to Squillante would do the trick, but again the question was why bother? Even if Jimmy and/or his pregnant girlfriend were round-the-bend nutso over the denial of their claims, stealing my company car a week later stretched credibility a little too thin.

Bill Eberly setting it up made slightly more sense, especially if he's connected to criminals whose power base requires quick and complete retribution for any personal harm, perceived or otherwise. Still I found it hard to imagine a gambler indebted to Squillante's bunch having the nerve to request the theft of a certain car. There was an agenda in play here I didn't quite get.

While reminding myself how clueless I still am, I drive to the Meadow Woods Shopping Center and parked in my favorite spot overlooking the Denmark Deli and Eberly Electronics. The hatchback is low and inconspicuous, and neither Tanner nor his uncle have any reason to connect it to me, so far as I know. A baseball cap and I'm as anonymous and I need to be.

The day is perfect for spying, clear and bright and cool, but I'm just not in the mood. I want to go watch Richard Kiel's house to get a better sense of him. Legwork and luck. Enough of the first and you get the latter.

As a precaution, I dial the Kiel residence on my borrowed cell phone hoping to learn whether Richard has a housekeeper or a live-in girlfriend. Amy's hallway was bad enough, but being the subject of two nine-one-one reports within twenty-four hours would be pushing my luck to the limit.

"I can't come to the phone right now," drones a recorded male voice.

I permit myself a satisfied smirk. Then I reach for the ignition.

Chapter 27

Richard Kiel's behemoth of a house is set on Drury Lane a discreet distance from the borderline of Landis. And what a tidy, opulent eyesore it is—a yellow block and brick two-story fronted by a sloping half-acre of professional landscaping so uninspired I want to yawn. Compounding the wasted excess, the neighboring custom-designed homes further what I call the cocktail party effect—everyone dressed up, but almost nobody has it right.

I park the hatchback past a curve in the street beside an enormous rhododendron, its leaves drawn in and dark from the cold. The neighborhood offers no sidewalks, so I pretend to be jogging until I reach Richard Kiel's mailbox. After a deep breath to settle my nerves, I turn into his driveway, which snakes uphill then plugs into a three-car garage spanning the whole right end of the house. Still jogging to stay warm, I stare at those three wide doors and try to talk myself out of breaking in.

I went through the same mental gymnastics regarding the East Side Pharmacy and decided it was a foolish risk—not because it would be wired tighter than a cockroach cage, because even if I was lucky enough to make off with an IV bag full of diluted drugs, it couldn't be used as evidence.

Two sets of books would be a slightly different story.

Drugs must be accounted for. Examiners expect whatever quantities a pharmacy buys wholesale to equal the inventory and sales exactly. And to satisfy the IRS, East Side's records damn well better match the company's reported income.

In other words, Richard would keep an accurate record of what he bought and sold, but he also needed to invent fake wholesale purchases and fake customers—and all the supporting paperwork—to account for the excess sales resulting from diluting the drugs.

Since businesses usually pay their suppliers by check, the fraudulent income would have to be run through the company account; but as sole proprietor, the profits would still end up in Kiel's pocket. An inflated tax bill would simply be the cost of doing business.

Me? I would hide the incriminating records at home where I could work on them at leisure and keep them safe from the prying eyes of my employees.

"Do no wrong," David lectured on my first day at AIA; and in that vague phrase I perceive just enough wiggle room to excuse what I'm about to do. If I'm lucky enough to nail Kiel for a crime, people will line up to thank me.

The house offers plenty of windows and doors, but I like what's right in front of me best—the horizontal row of square windows decorating the garage. They bring to mind the shoulder-high push-button switch just inside my parents' old garage door. Maybe this place will have one, too.

From the ugly pink edging along the front walk I select a rock the size of a softball. One last glance around and I saunter up to the far right window and give it a good smack. Shards of glass pop and fly and chime on the cement floor, but luckily I don't get cut. Leaving my DNA at the crime scene would be very bad karma.

I dry the nervous sweat off my forehead with the cuff of my sweatshirt then pull my hand inside the sleeve and knock out the rest of the glass with the rock.

And there it is—the switch I hoped for. Pressing it with smug satisfaction, I watch the door rise on well-greased runners, quickly close myself inside, turn around...and notice a blinking red security light up in the corner of the garage ceiling.

Damn.

Arm up over my face, I rush past an SUV, a barrel of athletic equipment, and some boxes. Up two steps I tug at the door to the house so hard I almost fall on my ass.

Stumble into the dining room–a blur of blue. Around the table. Through the kitchen into the laundry room. The security keypad is beside the back door—three rows of numbers set in a plastic square.

Birthday, the dummy's favorite code number. When the hell was Kiel's birthday? I read it in his bio...the year made him fifty-four. October 12! Frantically, I punch the numbers and hold my breath. Nothing happens.

Then I realize that silent alarms aren't supposed to warn the intruder; they alert the police.

I will my body to move, rubbing my itchy palms as I run. What else have I forgotten in my four years off the force? *The prearranged fail-safe.*

Alarms go off by mistake with maddening regularity, which is why the police often phone before they dispatch a squad car.

Okay, I'll pretend to be Kiel's ditzy girlfriend. "Sorry, fellas. Richard gave me the code, but I guess I got it wrong." Might buy me some time. Or it might not.

Richard Kiel's computer is in his first floor office, a bookish, leathery enclave of masculine efficiency. Using my sweatshirt cuff again, I press the on switch then head straight for the used rewriteable CDs in the plastic tower on the desk. Most people know that erased files can be retrieved by an expert, so finding anything incriminating on Kiel's hard drive seems unlikely. So as soon as the PC is up and running I sample a couple of the CDs to see if the labels match the material.

Unfortunately, "Investments" is clearly investments, and "Personal Mailing List" seems to be just that. "Recipes" and "Inventory" and "East Side" and "West Side" are all great temptations; but even though there's been no police check-in, I can't trust that I've disabled the alarm. I shut down the computer and look in his closet instead.

Sitting there big as life is a small safe, which I probably couldn't open if I had a month. The chances of the phony financial records being in there are probably only 50/50 anyhow. Why put your incriminating stuff in the first place the authorities would look? Me, I'd want them out where they would be easy to palm and discard.

What I'm really after is on the shelf with the rest of Kiel's office supplies—a new package of CD-RWs. I unwrap six, stuff the cellophane in my pocket and substitute the new, empty CDs for the labeled ones from the tower. Then I set about checking the drawers and bookcases for any interesting discs not out in plain sight.

Nada, but then what did I expect?

I hide the "West Side" disc behind a huge Merck Manual. Then on a whim I grab an old-fashioned leather-tipped ledger book from the shelf above and take it with me. I guess the symbolism appeals to me, the message. Mess with my mind, bozo, and I'll mess with yours.

In the dining room I yank out drawers full of polished silver, pressed linens, trivets. I hide another disc under an ecru tablecloth—"East Side," I think.

Still no check-in from the police, not a good sign unless my guess of the birthday code happened to be correct. Regardless, I'm not leaving until I'm good and ready.

The living room drawers contain the TV remote, assorted warranties and a nail file. I hide another CD down the left side of the sofa, a soft blue tapestry-patterned thing. Then I bound up the stairs. "Recipes" go under the guest room mattress—I say guest room because there are no clothes in the closet, no tissues or books or reading lamps anywhere.

Giving the master bedroom only a cursory glance—it gives me the creeps, to be honest—I run back down to the kitchen, where I hide the old ledger in among the cookbooks in a white, mullioned cabinet over the cutting board.

I make it to the front hallway and almost to the door before a man's voice freezes me in mid step. "Stop right there," it orders.

Not the official announcement.

I turn...slowly.

Civilian clothes. Murderous eyes. A gun between his hands. Apparently Richard Kiel called off the police so he could confront me himself.

Which tells me he's guilty. An innocent man would have left this to the pros.

Fury trumps my fear, and Beck stubbornness stiffens my spine. This man causes unthinkable suffering; and if he kills me, nobody else will stop him. Not now. Maybe not for years.

I have to get out of here alive. It's just that simple.

Stuck in the back of my waistband, my Glock is useless. All I can do is assess my captor with ice-cold calculation.

There's a chin aggressively thrust forward. Thin hard lips set in a frown. Pale eyebrows—arched. Trim physique. Taut, tanned face. Expensive clothes. All of which suggest excessive pride to me, possibly even conceit.

I have to be right—it's all I've got.

"Give me one good reason why I shouldn't kill you," he demands.

I extend my hands in the universal back-off gesture and ease a little closer to the door. "The police would be all over you," I tell him reasonably, "and you can't afford that."

Kiel laughs as he sidesteps the hall table. He's seen my back; he knows I can't get to the Glock. "Shooting an armed intruder? I'll take my chances."

This is how I'm going to die? After everything else, this is it?

"You're forgetting something," I blurt. "All that trouble you took—you wouldn't want to waste it, would you?"

Kiel's face twitches. "What the hell...?"

"My checking account, my credit card, my phone," I recite. "You've been a busy boy."

Hearing the list, something new dawns on me. "You gave me another reason to kill Corinne!"

"Really?" Said as if I were crazy.

"Money," I think out loud. "Either I couldn't stand to let her suffer, or I was desperate for an inheritance." Two very persuasive motives. Given those choices, no jury would believe a word out of my mouth. I'm not in her will, but I might have thought I was...

I tell Kiel, "I'm impressed." Intentional flattery, yes, but also true.

Of course framing me for murder wouldn't have been possible if Corinne survived.

"So how'd you do it?" I press. "A little something in her IV drip?" Any pharmacist would know a couple of poisons that don't show up in a post-mortem.

Kiel's eyes shift off center, allowing me a mere instant to lunge forward and give the gun a high kick.

A bullet hits the ceiling. The pistol falls and skitters out of reach.

Kiel curses and lashes out, but I hook his knees with my foot and sweep his legs out from under him. While he's still scrambling, I tug the door open and hurl myself out onto the lawn.

"Help, help," I shriek to the old woman opening her mailbox across the street. "There's a rapist in there!"

It's unlikely that Kiel will shoot me in front of a witness; but I keep hollering until I reach the hatchback, jump in, and fire it up.

Behind me the old woman waddles uphill, her mail scattered all around.

Chapter 28

Leaving Drury Lane and Richard Kiel behind, I drive with ferocious determination for ten minutes then pull over to the first available curb.

Heart pounding, I hammer the steering wheel and swear. Wipe away furious tears and blow my nose.

A couple more minutes of that and I decide enough already. I huff into my cold hands and look around, notice I'm in the middle of a split-level/swing-set neighborhood. On a fair-weather Tuesday I doubt that anybody will bother me, at least not right away.

Halfway down the block three junior-high boys climb out of a school bus. Backpacks over their puffy jackets, they pretend to dribble and pass a non-existent basketball, a scene so innocent and normal that I'm forced to remember that life is mostly good, that the Richard Kiels of the world are in the minority.

I take a deep breath and slowly let it out, deliberately reining myself in.

Yet as rationality takes over I begin to squirm. What if I'm not on the high road? What if I need to believe Corinne's death is a crime only because I want so desperately to avenge it?

I am compelled to make things right; that's why I became a cop. But back then I didn't wake up sobbing, and my insides never felt hollow all day. Just this morning I made up another joke for Corinne before I remembered she's gone, and the aftershock clenched my stomach into such knots that I thought I was going to be sick. So maybe I'm no stronger, no wiser, no braver, no less inclined to make mistakes than anybody else. Brent, for example. Was it possible that I'm just as wrong about Richard Kiel?

I replay today's confrontation in my head, from Kiel's "Give me one good reason why I shouldn't kill you" demand to his "What the hell...?" and realize that nothing the pharmacist said even remotely resembled an admission of guilt.

I don't even know whether the CDs I concealed around his house are incriminating. I only got to check a few before I had to hide the whole batch.

Then there was that eye shift, that little lapse of concentration that gave me my break. Kiel had looked confused. And why not? I had just accused him of murder.

Maybe I had better start over.

One more time: Who wants me down and out? No brainer. Nina, Nina, and Nina. Nobody else hates me quite so much.

Again, I might be wrong, but it occurs to me that there's a simple way to find out: Look her in the eye and ask her.

Putting Karen's hatchback in gear, I proceed directly to the house and park in the driveway. Through the kitchen window I see Nina speaking into the phone with her back turned to the door. The drab outfit she's wearing gives me a glimpse of her in ten or twenty years–still living in this house, still bitter and alone.

When I knock, she jumps and hastily hangs up.

"Let me in, Nina," I call through the door. "We need to talk."

She complies, but instead of her usual huffy greeting she folds her arms across her waist and shrinks away. Still, her focus feels predatory, so I ease my way in with caution.

Using my most soothing voice, I tell her that I'm sorry if I caused her any discomfort. "It's over—all of it. I'm ready to go away and leave you alone, but first there's something I need to ask..."

Nina's cheeks color, and her eyes flash. "You killed my mother and now you're back here trying to do what? Make peace?" An eerie laugh bubbles up from her chest. "Go to hell, Lauren." She has backed around the end of the kitchen island and rested her hand just above the knife drawer.

Fearful now, I hear her words but don't digest their meaning. "... *called the cops...can't get away with...*"

The kitchen door slams open, and suddenly Scarp Poletta is here pointing his gun–at me.

"Move away," he orders Nina before commanding me to turn around. "Hands on the wall where I can see them."

"What's going on?" I've retreated so fast and so far that I'm up against the cookie jars.

His partner covers me as Scarp pats me down for a weapon. It's repulsive, humiliating. I can smell his fresh sweat, feel his warm breath on my neck. As he snaps handcuffs around my wrists, he recites, "Lauren Beck, you're under arrest for the murder of Amy Dion. You have the right to remain silent. You have the right to an attorney..."

I don't hear the rest for the pounding in my head.

Did he say Amy? Amy Dion is dead?

Chapter 29

I am aware of Scarp pushing me into the squad car with his hand on my head, but mostly I'm too stunned to care what's happening.

Amy Dion is dead.

The car door slams at my side.

Amy, oh my, I'm so sorry. I should have found another way, but I set you on this course. I might as well have killed you myself.

The car begins to roll.

The tightness in my throat is unbearable, and sudden tears erupt. Holding back is impossible, so I let myself dissolve. Gasping sobs screw up my face and leave me sniveling and embarrassed. With my hands cuffed behind me I can't even clean myself up.

"You got a handkerchief up there?" I croak through the steel mesh to Scarp. He's riding shotgun, seething and staring out the window.

"No," he snaps without turning his head. From intimacy to total disgust in less than twenty-four hours. Incredible. Another straw for the camel's back.

I wipe my chin on my shoulder and watch the world rush by. Twilight is falling, and headlights dot thinner-than-usual afternoon traffic. We'll get to the Landis police station in record time.

I better hurry up and get a grip. Unless I can convince Scarp to keep an open mind, the police will stop looking for Amy's killer; and I certainly can't do it myself from jail.

"Listen," I say sharply enough to draw Scarp's attention. "I need to tell you something."

"Not now," he warns, as if I've forgotten about the driver.

"Yes, now," I persist. "You really need to hear this. Remember I said I went a little crazy on Amy and complained about Corinne's cancer treatment?"

"You have the right to remain *silent*..."

"What I really did was question whether the chemo drugs she got were full strength."

The veins in the detective's neck begin to bulge and throb.

"So when my life started falling apart, I asked Amy to ask the cancer registrar..."

Scarp wheels around, his face a dangerous red. "Will you please shut the fuck up?"

As predicted, we quickly arrive at the Landis Municipal Building, the city's primary facility and a far newer one than the care-worn Kynlyn Street sub-station. The Main, as it is called, also houses the tax collector and the mayor and animal control. But all of these are segregated from the police department's domain, which takes up the whole back end of the first floor with uptight newness and cold efficiency. I worked out of here a year, but I can honestly say that I never took to the place.

When Scarp was on the Landis force, he worked here, too; and apparently the county job still affords him local privileges because he dismisses his driver with a curt, "I'll take it from here."

We proceed past Dispatch into a roomful of desks, only half of which are occupied. I check around, anxious to see whether anybody I know is on duty—Garry Knutsen from the bar, for instance, or any of the others. I recognize a couple of faces, but I don't know anybody by name.

After a few words with the chief and some preliminary paperwork, Scarp delivers me to a locked room where a female cop performs the dreaded body search. Next, the flash of the mug-shot camera permanently etches the whole horrible episode into my brain.

Scarp and I aren't really face to face again until he moves my handcuffs from the back to the front for the fingerprint routine. Done on a console that's part computer and part Xerox machine, you sort of roll each fingertip on glass and photocopy it.

While he concentrates on getting a good thumb impression, I lean in to inquire discreetly, "Why me? Did Richard Kiel give me up, or what?"

No eye contact.

"Kiel, right?" I press. "Or was it some anonymous *man*?"

Scarp finishes rolling my thumb before he gives in to temptation. "You broke into his house. What did you expect him to do?"

Denial will sound like a lie and so will an evasion, so I re-script the truth. "All I did was throw a rock through his window...to...get him to come out."

The detective winces and rolls his eyes. "You ever hear of knocking on somebody's door?"

"I did that. Then I rattled it, and the silent alarm must have gone off because Kiel came home almost right away. The trouble was he went in the back and I missed him. So I..."

"... broke his garage window with a rock."

"Yes. I needed to talk to him." And that is why our mothers warn us not to take that treacherous path. One lie leads to another which leads to another, and so on and so on until you're lost.

"So did you?"

"What?"

"Talk to him."

"Yes. No. Yes."

"You really shouldn't be telling me any of this."

"You're going to find out anyhow."

Poletta glances around the squad room. Five officers are working at desks, two speaking to each other. No one is giving us much more than an infrequent glance, so Scarp leans forward and prompts, "What really happened?"

I ease a little closer, too. "I sort of told Kiel I thought he was responsible for Corinne's death."

"You think he killed her?"

"Well, no. Not anymore."

Scarp nods. "Good. That's good. Because the hospital personnel have been over Corinne's records with us upside-down and backward," he remarks almost casually, "and nobody found one shred of evidence to support a charge of murder."

"Thanks for telling me now."

"I would have gotten around to it."

I want to know more about Amy, but I need to be careful what I say. When the fingerprinting business is done, I ask to use the rest room.

Scarp escorts me as far as the door. Then he stands there for a moment just looking at me, his eyes so distant that it hurts.

"I didn't kill anybody," a desperate cliché, but I can't help myself.

"Your company car was found two blocks from Amy's apartment," Poletta informs me with what appears to be regret. "And you were seen brandishing a gun outside her door. The press will run the D.A. out of town if he doesn't indict you."

"But you know I didn't do it. I was with you!"

Scarp shakes his head. "I don't know any such thing, Lauren. You took off from my place right after dinner, remember? Do you deny that you went to Amy's before you came back?"

So the woman from the hall came forward, the one who caught me shouting at Amy with a gun in my hand. I slump against the wall and might have slid right on down to the floor if Scarp hadn't grabbed my shoulders.

"Amy was Corinne's nurse, right?" he reminds me. "So the prosecution will argue that you blamed her for Corinne's death." He shakes his head. "You're gonna need a miracle to get out of this."

"Will you help me?"

Scarp just stares. "I can only do my job, Lauren. No more and no less."

I ought to try to talking him around, but I don't have the strength.

"Go wash up." He turns me toward the door then opens it.

I stagger into the empty women's room—familiar black and white tile, a row of sinks and a row of enclosed toilets, one daybed, and two towel holders. Nothing a desperate woman could use to harm herself or anyone else. Even the mirror is made of steel.

I spend a couple of minutes feeling sorry for myself and a couple more bitching under my breath before I suck it up and wash my hands and face.

The work area outside the holding cell has a desk with a phone. Scarp picks up the receiver and offers it to me. One call and only one, so I know it had better count.

"Not yet," I decide.

The detective's eyebrows rise, but all he says is, "Give Tim here a holler when you're ready." Then he turns tail and aims for the door.

I wanted to say, "Be careful out there," but I would have been talking to myself.

Examining the holding cell takes less than a second; there is a shelf-like bench attached to a wall surrounded by bars. Period. Being an interior room, it doesn't even own a window, just a view of the small processing area and the end of the squad room that contains one unoccupied desk. Tim, my cop babysitter, sits at a nearby table and fiddles around with a computer.

Perched on the shelf, I pull my knees up to my chest and think about getting myself out of here. A key ingredient, so to speak, is that all-important phone call, so I take my good old time rehearsing for that. Finally, I shout to the guard that I'm ready.

"Need me to look up your lawyer's number?" he offers. His reading glasses are dirty and he has a cold, but there is no mistaking the authority in his stance.

"No thanks." I know the number I want by heart. Office hours are ending, but my oncologist is a widower and hates to go home.

"Here, take my chair." Tim gestures with his left hand while his right rests on his gun.

I tell him, "Thanks," but then warn him that it may take a while.

Forty minutes to be precise, fifteen for Dr. Shrawder to come to the phone then twenty-five for me to outline what I need. The cancer specialist isn't used to this sort of emergency, but to his credit he listens with undivided attention then agrees to do what I ask as soon as humanly possible.

"I have patients," he reminds me unnecessarily, since, if checkups count, I'm still one of them.

"I do, too," I reply, and my elderly oncologist musters up a polite laugh.

I express my gratitude and tell the dear doctor good-bye.

For about a minute I congratulate myself on how wise I was to call him.

Then the cell door closes behind me, and my confidence flees.

Have I just wasted my one and only call?

Chapter 30

Rush hour came and went, and the shifts changed. Now my babysitter is an officer named Jacob Yeager, which, close as we are to Amish country, makes him sound more like a pacifist than a peacekeeper.

"Dinner," he announces, unceremoniously handing me a bag from Burger King.

I flick the salt off the first French fry, but then just eat by instinct.

Richard Kiel killed Amy; I'm as sure of that as I am of my own name. He is the evil monster the oncology nurse and I shuddered to imagine, a person so arrogant and immoral that he can dilute chemotherapy drugs for profit and still sleep at night.

As much as I appreciated Scarp's warning about Bill Eberly's connections, I never managed to summon up a healthy fear of the guy. He comes across as a blustery playground bully, the sort you don't want to cross, but identity theft? premeditated auto theft? He just isn't that evolved.

Jimmy Tanner? A wannabe thug at best, his threats no different from the ones I heard every day as a cop. Although he probably did borrow a pickup to follow me home from the hospital; he's that kind of pain in the ass.

Bob Battersby? With no connection to Amy, a neurotic jerk but nothing more.

I finish my dinner and wad up the wrapper. Shoot it at the trashcan and miss.

Yeager's feet are up, and he's working his way through the *Philadelphia Inquirer*. Even from my cell I can read the three-inch headline about the murder.

"Hey," I call over. "Borrow that when you're through?"

Yeager checks around for his boss then slips the front section through the bars.

The article is pretty short on facts, but I do learn more about my stolen company car. Apparently I abandoned it because of—imagine the odds—a flat tire.

The murder method is one of the omissions, but I have my own idea about that. A lethal drug requires premeditation—not a given—and I can't imagine a nurse falling for something like that. A gunshot would have roused the neighbors instantly, and strangulation isn't as easy as it sounds. I put my money on the ever-popular blunt instrument—handy, silent, and sure.

Trading sections with Yeager one at a time, I manage to relieve my mind about Kathy Parker. The cancer registrar's name isn't mentioned, perhaps because she insisted that no tampering occurred, a conviction that supports Kiel rather than threatens him. Also, reversing her position would suggest that she failed at her job, an admission she was unlikely to make. Bottom line: For Kiel, leaving Kathy alone was the safer choice.

About seven the attorney I asked Dr. Shrawder to contact on my behalf arrived. As a cop, I was familiar with all the criminal lawyers in town, so it was just a matter of picking an appropriate one off my mental list. Arabella Johnson got the nod because she's smart, female, and black, which always seems to unsettle the Assistant District Attorneys she comes up against. Plus she's as tenacious as a bad rash and hates stupidity almost as much as she hates injustice. At least that's her reputation. We're meeting for the first time.

"Got ourselves in a bit of a bind, do we?" she says, offering her warm hand after Yeager closes the door of the private meeting room behind us. Five feet four and broad of beam, she wears her dense black hair braided around the top of her head. The glasses perched on her broad nose are also thick and black, contrasting only slightly with her rich sienna skin. Her expression seems more calculating than friendly, but I don't mind. My job is to win her over, not the other way around.

"Not me," I answer. "But I think the cops do."

"Oh?" she responds, her right eyebrow arched with curiosity. "Let's hear it."

I fill her in on the cast of characters and how I came to be arrested.

Then I say, "I didn't do it," and watch ennui shroud her face. *Tell me something I don't hear every day*, her demeanor begs. So I do.

I begin with the outburst in the hallway at Soames and how it must have terrified Richard Kiel right down to his socks. "Lucky for him, I was crazed with grief, or he would have had to kill me."

The eyebrow twitches, so I explain that making me appear even more desperate and unstable leaves Kiel's insulation intact. Until Amy, he performed all his mayhem at arm's length.

"Also, he's no dope," I add. "When people die, other people ask questions."

Arabella maintains an encouraging silence, so I continue to blame all my troubles on Richard Kiel. My favorite arguments: convincing Nina that I'm responsible for her mother's death and phoning the police to frame me for Amy.

Throughout, Arabella comports herself like a benevolent mother figure, one who isn't easily fooled. Unfortunately, the more I talk the more I begin to worry that my lawyer doesn't give a damn about me.

"Hey," I shout at one point. "Are you paying attention?"

Ignoring that, she says, "Tell me about Amy."

Feeling as if I'm running in place, I talk faster. "I doubt that her murder was premeditated. I think Kiel just wanted to see where she stood, maybe bad-mouth me in person." Somebody certainly did. "Maybe he took his pharmacist flunkie along to help him get in the door—maybe not. But one thing's for sure. Amy couldn't hide her feelings from a blind man. It would have been obvious to Kiel that she didn't trust him, and that meant she had to go."

"Sorry," my attorney says with a flurry of blinks, "why wouldn't she trust him?"

I huff and fidget.

"The printouts," I reply with a sigh. "After our lunch, Amy probably found something in the statistics that tipped her off to the fraud. Maybe she even realized—as I finally did—that Kiel stayed under the cancer registrar's radar by diluting the drugs at random." With patience and discipline, he could gather nest eggs for years to come.

I also think Kiel's in-house confidante, Sara, probably saw Amy and me with our heads together—very bad news for a nervous crook. To split us up, Kiel, either personally or through Sara, put the bug in Amy's ear about me, tightening the frame already in place regarding Corinne. The result: Amy turned me away and gave the pharmacist a brief reprieve.

Brief, because his worst fear now had teeth. My chance remark was being pursued—by me, and by a reputable oncology nurse. Me, the persona non grata, he could deal with later; but with Amy onto the fraud, he had to act fast, before she could involve the authorities.

After I finish my pitch, Arabella describes the arraignment formality—as if I didn't know—then rises and delicately taps the door with her knuckles. I probably look like the guy on the island who just cast another plea for help into the ocean.

Sensing my eyes on her back, Arabella pauses long enough to say, "See you in the morning."

"Bring breakfast," I suggest, only half joking.

A tolerant grunt and the woman is gone.

In the morning, she promised. So she either believes me or likes the challenge of my case. I'm too numb to either cheer or cry with relief; but I think I may be able to sleep later on, and that's progress enough for now.

However, Yeager and a partner first have to transport me by car to Glendenning County Correctional. It seems that my new lawyer arranged to save herself a trip out into the countryside. Nice. A woman with clout. And still Scarp's "You're gonna need a miracle to get out of this" keeps circling around in my head.

GCC is a prison, what else can I say? The steel doors lock with that resounding thunk—the live version of dirt hitting the lid of your coffin. But here at least the cells offer niceties such as running water and bedding, the reason why I couldn't stay overnight in the Landis lockup.

Being an ex-cop, I've been put in a private accommodation segregated from the rest of the women serving time. You never know when an inmate is holding a giant grudge, and some of them remain guests of the state for a long long while. In a way I'm glad for the solitude.

I sleep some. Not much. I can hear other distant inmates fussing and fuming through the walls. Plus my cot isn't actually conducive to rest.

In the morning they hustle me off to District Court where I meet up again with Arabella. When our turn comes, the judge launches into his, "Lauren Beck, you are charged with murder in the first degree blah, blah, blah. How do you plead?" I answer, "Not guilty, your honor," and that's about it. There isn't much of a discussion about bail because it's a capital offense and I'm not eligible. "Maybe later," Arabella whispers out of the side of her mouth when she sees me begin to tremble.

Scarp sits in the first row of spectators—did I mention the horde of reporters?—and I manage to throw a "Speak to you?" over my shoulder on my way out.

He catches up with me and my transport team in the alley behind the courthouse.

"A favor?" I begin when the officers pause at his request. "My laptop?" My incarceration is looking to be more onerous than I expected, and I need a serious distraction to help me wait out Dr. Shrawder's research assignment. Writing down the series of events that got me locked up sounds like just the ticket; so I'm counting heavily on Scarp to come through, probably way more than our brief relationship deserves.

His dark eyes bulge with disbelief, and I think he may actually sputter.

"Why?" he finally manages.

Meanwhile, the officers have caught on that this isn't an important police matter and are man-handling me into the cop car. "Type my confession," I fib for their benefit.

Hands on his hips, Scarp shakes his head as we pull away.

Chapter 31

Apparently Scarp was able to do something with the "Type my confession" remark, because he just arrived with my laptop. I noticed that he entrusted the overnight charger/cord to the matron on his way in just in case I'm feeling suicidal. Also, my cell has no electrical outlet, something I hadn't considered.

Scarp is sitting beside me on the lower bunk, not too close and not too far. Neither of us quite knows what to say.

"Thanks for pulling strings," I finally tell him as evenly as I can. "I would go crazy in here without something to do." Something of an understatement.

Scarp shrug that off. "The boss thinks it'll make for interesting reading."

I don't bother to smile. "You're really taking some chances with your career for me," I remark. "Thanks."

"You didn't do it, did you?"

"No."

"Then I'm not taking much of a chance."

Still, the man seems a bit angry for some reason. Best to wait that out.

"I need to know a couple things, Lauren," he finally begins, "and no bullshit this time."

I nod. He deserves my best behavior. Always has, I guess, but I didn't trust myself completely, so I held back.

"Were you ever inside Amy's apartment?"

"No, I wasn't. She wouldn't let me in."

"Keep talking."

"She'd invited me to stay with her—that's why I went. That and I wanted to see the printouts she brought home from Soames."

"Go on."

"Nobody answered my knock. I used the extra key Amy told me about, but she had the chain bolt on. That's when I found out she was in there alone, scared to death—of me."

"Alone?"

"If she had a friend with her, she wouldn't have sounded so skittish. Two against one, you know? And if somebody else was there and she was afraid of them, I think I would have detected some excitement in her voice. After all, I was coming to the rescue, right?"

"Reasonable. So what changed? Why suddenly become afraid of you?"

"Had to be Kiel or his friendly little confidante putting the bug in her ear. Saying I really did kill Corinne, something like that. Doesn't matter, I guess. Bottom line—she never let me in."

"You put the key back?"

"I must have. It wasn't in the stuff you inventoried yesterday."

"Now explain about the gun."

"I was jumpy—everything that's been going on, your warning about Squillante. I heard a noise in the hall behind me and took it out. Then I got talking to Amy and I guess I never put it away."

"*Arguing* with Amy." It isn't a question.

I shrug. No denying how it sounded to someone else.

All Scarp did was stand up, but suddenly it feels as if he's blocks away, maybe miles.

"So then you came over and shacked up with me," he says, hitching his thumb behind his belt. "How convenient for you. A bed *and* an alibi."

I can tell that I've blanched, but I scramble to my feet thinking maybe I ought to defend myself. Yet there is no quick way to explain my insecurities, so simply say, "It wasn't like that at all."

"You used me, Lauren. Do you deny it?"

"Would you believe me if I did?"

He sucks his cheek and rocks back on his heels. "No, I guess not."

"May I still have the computer?" I ask a little desperately as he signals to be let out of my cell.

I'm sure he would love to deprive me of my one special privilege, but to his credit he just lifts his chin and levels his eyes. "Like I said, my boss wants to see what you have to say."

"You don't?"

"Me?" he replies. "I got better things to do."

After a soggy BLT and a carton of orange juice for lunch, I start my chronicle of this whole mess at the beginning, October 29, the day I was offered the job with Amalgamated.

The battery hangs in all the way up to my first interview with Megan DeMarquess at the recycling plant, which was also the day our household mail went missing. Getting the matron's attention requires a lot of yelling and stomping, but eventually she saunters in.

"Can you please recharge this?" I request as nicely as I know how.

The woman, the female version of a fireplug with a knot of thinning hair, throws me a look so scathing that I fear I'll never see my computer again.

"The D.A. is waiting for me to type my confession," I call after her, because unfortunately, it's the truth. "Check it out if you don't believe me."

The woman must have done exactly that, because about an hour and a half later she returned with the laptop all charged up and ready to go. I'd dozed off waiting, and the clang of the metal outer door sent my heart into a frenzy.

"Thanks," I manage to mumble, then wake up enough to beg, "Please clear this with the next shift? I think I'm gonna be up all night."

The woman shot me a scowl and a snort that, were she a guy, would have been a spit. Yet the D.A. connection must have done the trick, because the next time the battery quit—just as my golf-club victim victory was leading into Corinne's pneumonia—the matron's nighttime equivalent complied without a squawk.

Such was my pattern for approximately thirty-seven hours—type until my hands ached and the battery warning blinked. Sleep. Type. Sleep. An extension cord would have been a huge help, but this is prison after all and deprivation was the whole point. I felt like a caterpillar in a chrysalis working my ass off trying to get out. To top off the depressing effect of my environment, it rained all Thursday; so the thin light eking through the high windows above the short row of cells might as well have been street lamps. I about went crazy trying to distract myself enough not to go crazy. It's been like having a fever so high and all consuming that afterward you regard it as separate from the rest of your year, a time when you're not living your life but are merely enduring it.

On the bright side, I had no time to obsess about what Dr. Shrawder was or was not learning about Richard Kiel.

I just pushed on, through Corinne's funeral and Norman Schmidt's alcoholism, through the demeaning day at the bank and Dennis Arquette's misinformed daughter. The healing visit with my brother, Bill Eberly's connection to Morris Squillante, and Scarp's warnings about them both; and yes, Scarp himself and our problematical one-night stand.

All the while I kept a tight lid on a seething fury, afraid of what might happen if I acknowledge just how much I hate Richard Kiel. Physical confinement is nothing compared to the emotions I've kept locked inside myself.

I'm not sure, but I think this is Friday morning. The original matron just woke me.

"Freshen up," she says. "You've got a meeting with Detective Poletta and a Doctor somebody with an S."

"What time is it," I croak.

"Nine-thirty. Hurry it up."

Exhilaration and dread course through me like a power surge, and when I've been delivered to a World War One style meeting room a short ten minutes later, my nerves are tingling. My face is scrubbed, but there was no time to comb my hair. At the sight of me Scarp's lips tighten into a brief, unfair grimace.

"Hello," I greet Dr. Shrawder.

"Please have a seat," the oncologist offers, as if sweeping the weight of responsibility right out from under me. Scarp settles at the opposite end of the table and holds himself so silent and still as to be almost invisible.

The thing I always notice first about my cancer specialist is his hands. Spare and long, they belong to a man evaporating with age. He also wears reading glasses, I know, cheap drug store ones framed in red or blue flecked with aqua. At an appointment you're so acutely aware of the colors that you overlook his wet gray eyes. Unadorned today, they expose a sorrow rooted deep in his core. During all the dark dark days of my disease, he remained consistently proficient and upbeat. Seeing him now, my palms begin to sweat.

"I got the court order you recommended." I'd worried that Kiel would use his connections to alter Soames's cancer records before Shrawder could study them.

"And?"

"You were right," he admits with a shallow sigh. "Lord knows it pains me to say it, but you were right."

I can't speak. My fingers twine into my hair and hold tight. My eyes fill with tears. Scarp slides me his handkerchief this time, and the two men wait while I use it and catch my breath.

"Please explain," I finally manage to ask.

Shrawder nods. "At first I limited my study to the charts of all the cancer patients Soames lost this year," he begins. "Some, but not all, showed unexpected irregularities in their blood counts during the course of their chemotherapy."

"What kind of unexpected irregularities?"

"As you know, when patients are on chemo their blood counts fall—without fail. It's a natural consequence of the treatment. When I began to study Soames's patients as a group, I looked for—and found—patients whose blood counts did not drop immediately after receiving their regular treatment."

"Why didn't anybody notice this before?"

"Because, as you suggested, the drugs were diluted at random." At this the doctor's face flushes with shame. "I suppose the patients were delighted by how well they felt, and the doctors—myself included, I'm sorry to say— simply judged the blood counts to be aberrations or the test too premature. Your criminal was very wise to keep his greed in check. If not for you, there's no telling how many patients he might have swindled out of their last chance for survival."

"So do we have him? Is it enough for an arrest?" I glance from the oncologist to Scarp and back.

Shrawder answers. "What I've mentioned is only part of what I did. After I determined that there was a possibility of tampering—and you have to understand that my initial review only represented a possibility—I broadened the scope. I did a computer search of all the cancer patients for the past year, concentrating on their blood counts. I charted my notes, and a pattern began to emerge—certain time spans when the drugs appeared to be ineffective. Those periods were defined well enough to suggest that the diluted drugs had been administered during the course of a week or two, the typical length of time before we reorder.

"As you might imagine, my concern became an obsession. I asked two of my assistants to work overnight with me to review all the records for the past five years—the duration of Soames's contract with East Side Pharmacy. And, yes, now that I have the results of that combined effort, I am prepared to testify under oath that the tampering did in fact occur."

I glance at Scarp. "You're not ready to make an arrest," I state because I already know he has a problem.

Scarp shifts his shoulders in that way I find so attractive, except this time he's not showing off. This time he's really squirming. "You know and I know that Kiel did the fraud—he's the only one who would profit from it—but we still don't have anything that says he's the guy and nobody else."

"But you have probable cause now, right? You can get a search warrant."

"Oh, yeah. We'll be looking to match up some trace material from Amy's apartment—fiber samples, hair and whatnot—and of course we've got our lab checking whether Soames's last batch of chemo drugs from East Side was diluted."

"It won't be," Shrawder laments.

"...but to wrap this up really tight," the county detective continues almost to himself, "I'd really love to get my hands on Kiel's books. He's gotta have two sets stashed somewhere—one to satisfy the drug regulators and another to support the excess profits for the IRS."

Exactly what I was thinking when I broke into Kiel's house, but since my search was illegal, I hid the suspicious discs so they could be discovered properly and used in court. If I got lucky and Kiel thought I stole them (and he didn't come across any accidentally), Scarp's legal search will give the D.A. all he needs to fry the slimy bastard. I would dearly love to take Scarp by the collar and personally lead him to the evidence, but of course–*I can't.*

"And you came here first because...?"

"Waiting on the warrant," Scarp replies. "Should be ready," a glance at his watch, "any minute now."

We lock eyes, but not for long. "So scram already," I tell him.

"You're okay for a while longer?"

"Oh, yeah," I lie. "I'm still working on my confession."

My oncologist shoots Scarp a puzzled look, but the detective just rolls his eyes. "Let's go, Doc," he tells Shrawder. "We're finished here."

I reach across the table to give the doctor's hand a warm squeeze. "Thanks," I tell him, "for everything."

He lowers his eyes and says, "You deserve all the credit."

Scarp hangs back to let the older man exit first, and as the prison matron resumes her responsibility for me, he remarks, "You're a piece of work, Beck, you know that?"

I nod. "Just keep me in the loop, will you?"

About three that afternoon, I'm lying down, staring at the underside of the top bunk and facing my feelings about Richard Kiel—at last. I suppose Shrawder's proof finally gave me permission. So lost am I in punishing the sick bastard that the snick of the metal outer door being unlocked shoots me upright.

Scarp, already back with news. "Well?"

He waits until we're locked in together before he replies.

"Nothing financial in Kiel's safe," he reports. "Nothing on his hard drive or on any of the discs we found anywhere near his computer."

"But you found the books anyway, right? Tell me you found them anyway."

Scarp makes a show of looking mildly curious. "You sure you didn't make it inside Kiel's house?"

"Why?"

"Because Kiel's backup discs were inside the cover of an old ledger stashed between *The Galloping Gourmet* and Julia Child."

"Are my prints on them or something?"

"No, but did you have to be so obvious? Cooked books! Jeez, Lauren. How corny can you get?"

I actually hadn't thought of that. "So am I out of here, or what?"

Scarp and I are seated on the bunk again. Now he drops his hands between his knees and slumps down toward them, obviously sorry as hell to let me down.

"Matching up the trace samples from Amy's with what we got at Kiel's will take time," he says. "I'm sorry, but..."

I know he'll tell me I'm stuck here until they have positive proof that Kiel was in Amy's apartment and that I was not, but I interrupt him.

"What did you say was in Kiel's safe?"

"No financial records. Just some cash, a watch, and a couple of computer discs that didn't pan out."

"Your guys use gloves when they touched the stuff?"

"Of course."

"Did one disc have something to do with Christmas?"

Scarp blinks. "Yes, but the tech checked, and it wasn't what we were after..."

"Yeah, but I bet it wasn't anybody's Christmas card list either."

"What are you getting at?"

"Just in case, I had Amy label the disc she got from the Soames's cancer registrar 'Christmas card list,' but I guess Kiel wasn't fooled. Or maybe Amy left it in her computer where it was a little too easy to find. Who knows? There was a printout, too, but that's probably confetti by now." I wave my head with regret. "Anyway, the disc came from Amy's apartment."

Scarp cocks his head and grins at me. "You really are a piece of work."

"Forgive me?" I ask, trying to capitalize on the grin.

Scarp stands and calls out for the matron before he answers. "Why don't we talk about that when you're out of here?"

An outright "yes" might have been nice, but I'm in no position to quibble.

"Sure," I tell him affably. "Let's go.

Chapter 32

Unfortunately, I was joking when I told Scarp, "Let's go." Legal machinery never operates quite that fast.

First he had to verify that the "Christmas card list" CD was indeed the same one Amy received from her friend Kathy. Since discs are usually handled by the edges, nobody expected any fingerprints and none were found. However, Scarp took a handwriting expert through the crime scene, and she matched the CD's hand-printed label with the printing on some storage boxes from Amy's closet.

Next came a positive I.D. from the cancer registrar, who was found having one helluva Friday night—watching TV in her socks and pajamas with a Lean Cuisine on her lap. She confirmed that the disc, minus the label, was identical to the one she prepared for Amy at my request. Scarp had his smoking gun; and, in theory, I had my freedom.

But not until Scarp's boss, the District Attorney who originally approved the criminal complaint against me, presented the new evidence to the county common pleas court judge assigned to my case so *he* could withdraw the charges.

Scarp was considerate enough to deliver the paperwork personally, and now it's ten after ten on Saturday morning and I'm breathing in crisp November air under the sunny skies outside of Glendenning County Correctional. My rescuer's beard is two days dense and his eyes a decade older than when he whisked me away from Corinne's funeral, reminding me that—to him—securing my freedom was a pretty low priority. And yet he did it.

"Thanks," I say as my breath freezes in front of my face. "You've gone out of your way." An understatement.

"Thought I owed you that," he responds, opening the passenger door of his work-worn county vehicle for me to climb in.

"Where to?" he inquires after he settles behind the wheel.

My eyes stray toward the razor-wire and the stone walls of the prison. "Away from here. That's for sure."

"Lauren," the homicide detective urges. "Pick somewhere. Anywhere. I gotta get back to work."

The trouble is I have nowhere to go. And when I open my mouth to point that out, nothing comes forth but air.

"Oh, shit," Scarp remarks with a sad wave of his head. "I forgot."

"I'm sorry. I just..."

"Never mind. Leave it to me." He checks the road behind us then pulls onto the two-lane. The surrounding fallow fields and empty trees of the countryside soothe my frayed edges and, naturally, make me think of Dad.

"What?" Scarp asks with the helpless dismay of a man saddled with a woman verging on tears.

"I know it's silly, but I miss my father."

"You've been through a lot."

"Yes," I agree. Another understatement.

"Here." Scarp pulls his cell phone off his belt and hands it to me.

"He's in Albuquerque," I remind him.

"Knock yourself out."

"Thanks."

I give myself a minute to stop sniveling, and then I dial.

For once, it's Dad who answers.

"Hey, Jellybean. How are ya?" he says when he hears my voice.

I struggle to sound light. "Hangin' in there. How about you?"

"Annie has me on a diet."

We toss that topic around a bit as if we have nothing more weighty to discuss. I even try to laugh, but it's no use. The question I've been dying to ask for months is like a sheet of rain in front of my face.

"There's something on my mind," I warn.

"Thought so. Go ahead."

I draw in a breath as if it were courage. "Why didn't you ask Corinne to marry you, Dad? Everybody thought you would."

After a beat, he says, "What makes you think I didn't?"

"Wha...waitaminute. You're saying you did?"

"Of course. The outcome wasn't anything to brag about, and anyhow I figured you'd hear it from Corinne..."

"No. No, she didn't tell me."

"Oh. Well, water under the bridge..."

"She turned you down?"

"Yup. That's about it."

It wasn't, not by a long shot. I'd been thinking ill of him–my own father–for no reason. For months he'd been at the top of my shit list right next to Brent W. Cahill, the selfish, cold-hearted ex-love of my life.

"Jeez, Dad. I am so sorry."

"Yeh, me too."

For a moment silence fills the space between us, until I confess, "I don't understand it. Why...?"

"I agree," Dad interjects. "I know why, but it still doesn't make any sense."

"What did she say?"

"That she couldn't stand to watch herself die through my eyes."

"Oh." It's not much of a reply, but it's all I can manage. We were in the same club, Dad and me. A lot to absorb. A lot to talk about.

However, Scarp has stopped the car, and the relative silence makes me look around. We are in Nina's driveway.

"Listen, Dad," I tell him. "I'd like to talk more, but I'll have to call back. Okay?"

"You bet, Jellybean. Later."

"Later," for sure. I press the Off button and return Scarp's phone.

"What's this?" I ask with a wave of my hand, but my escort is already getting out of the car.

"Leave the talking to me," he advises. "But can we hurry it up? I..."

"...gotta get back to work," I finish for him.

Scarp knocks on the kitchen door, rocking on his heels and nodding reassurance while we wait.

Nina responds with a basket of towels on her hip. Her clean, Saturday-morning face reminds me of Corinne when she was ill.

"We would like to come in," Scarp announces, flashing his shield to indicate that this is police business.

"What's she doing here?" Nina demands, but Scarp halts her with his hand.

After securing the door behind us, he addresses Corinne's daughter with grave formality. "It is my understanding that you evicted your tenant, Ms. Beck here, without warning and without cause, and I would like you to correct that."

Nina sets the basket on the counter and her hand on her hip. "Oh, you would, huh?" she says. "I'm supposed to let a murderer live under the same roof as me and my daughter? What's she doing out of jail anyway?"

Scarp doesn't have time for an argument. He straightens to his full height. "The charges against Ms. Beck have been dropped. The county has determined that she is innocent, and she's been released with our apologies."

"Innocent, huh?" Nina gives me one of her patented looks, and I know she's still thinking about me and her mother.

The implication is not lost on Scarp. "I'm sure when you've had time to reconsider what happened, you'll realize that Ms. Beck is as much a victim of an opportunistic criminal as you were. Perhaps then you can..."

"Ms. Beck knows what I think."

Scarp looks as if he's about to try one of those now-girls phrases, but he sees my face and opts for the legal argument.

"Okay," he says. "You," he refers to Nina, "will serve Ms. Beck with a proper termination notice that gives her ample time to find another accommodation. And you," he means me, "will make every effort to comply. Now I really must get back to work. Ladies, I trust we're both alright here?"

Nina and I grunt in unison.

"Good." He takes his leave, slamming the door and not looking back.

"I'll pay you," I tell Nina as I tug the door back open.

I think she said, "You won't be here that long," but I'm already outside trying to catch up with Scarp.

He's getting into his car, so I shout, "Why the rush?" It has finally occurred to me that if Richard Kiel were in custody, the lead detective would have been breathing easier. The fact that he wasn't meant that Amy's killer was still at large, something I might have figured out sooner if I hadn't been so self-absorbed.

The face Scarp turns toward me says it all.

I lift my eyes to the sky and swear. Then I spin around and swear some more.

"Sorry," I finally apologize.

"No. No, you're right. We're a bunch of fucking incompetents."

"I was cursing Richard Kiel. But forget about that. Tell me what happened."

We began to walk toward the street, to keep warm and to relieve some stress. We stop at the sidewalk and face each other.

Scarp waves his head. "We couldn't find him, Lauren. Not at the pharmacy, not at his home. We put out an all-points bulletin, and all that got us was his car—in the long-term parking lot at Philly International."

"But all that security! How could he possibly fly anywhere without getting caught?"

The detective looks miserable. "We're not ruling out anything yet," he tells me. "While we're checking flights we're also watching buses and trains. Every squad car has his picture plastered to the dashboard. Hell, the whole country knows we're looking for the sonovabitch. We'll get him, don't worry."

It's all a bit overwhelming. Scarp had been going through hell during the last sixteen hours, but he still fit in the bookkeeping chores that got me out of jail. I felt honored, but I also felt awful. If Kiel had an eye on the cancer registrar's place, or Amy's apartment, or the judge, he might have fled because he picked up on the process of my release.

"What can I do to help?"

"Nothing, Lauren. We'll take it from here. Really. Don't worry about it."

"Don't worry about it? Don't worry about it! I get harassed all to hell and thrown in jail, and now you want me to stay home and play house? Think again, buster."

"Com'on, Lauren. You know what I mean. You're out of the business. There isn't anything you can do."

I wrap my arms around myself as if that will contain my anger. "What about the ex-wife? I've been having great luck with ex-wives lately. What about her?"

"Dead end, Lauren. She remarried and moved away. We don't even know her name."

"Then you won't mind if I try to find her, right?"

"What the hell, sure. But you get anything, you bring it straight to me." He waits while I absorb the non-verbal portion of the message. *You're personally involved,* his eyes warn. *Leave this to the professionals.*

"Absolutely," I agree, not because I don't trust myself, because I have no authority to arrest Kiel even if I find him.

Still, it's the answer Scarp wants to hear. Lauren Beck will not be underfoot; she will be safely off in cyberspace chasing after a phantom. He gives me a pat on the back and steers me toward the kitchen door. "Keep in touch," he says a little too heartily.

"You, too," I reply with a satisfied smile of my own.

True, the avenues the police are pursuing probably stand the best chance of capturing Kiel, but I'm not exactly going to be tilting at windmills. Considering how I've been earning my living for the past four years, I like my chances of finding the ex-wife.

I like them a lot.

Chapter 33

Scarp speeds off in a cloud of exhaust, and I go back inside. That's when I notice that the bobbleheads and cookie jars are gone; only the shelves remain. Like a physical blow, it hits me that I no longer want to be here, not without Corinne's music and Corinne's friendship and Corinne's things. If I weren't on a mission, I'd go upstairs and pack the rest of my belongings here and now.

Corinne and then Amy. And now Richard Kiel is on the run. More than anything I want to bring him down myself, to cuff him and read him his rights and watch his arrogance die. But I know that isn't going to happen. I'm lucky Scarp agreed to let me participate at all. Very lucky.

Ignoring the mess that is my apartment, I retrieve my laptop from my duffel bag and set it back on its table in the southern dormer.

Within five minutes I'm reviewing Richard Kiel's vital statistics—every address past and present, his neighbors' names, all phones linked to him including cell phones and unlisted numbers, every property, every loan including co-signers, all his vehicles and their identification numbers, and of course that 45-foot sailboat. I hope the fact that he retained all that stuff still annoys his ex-wife. The more disgruntled the spouse, the more eager she will be to dish the dirt.

Her first name is Anne, and during the past year Richard signed over two apartment buildings to her. The ownership of another, smaller, rental property was also switched to him alone. Odds were that plenty of cash also changed hands to settle the divorce, but financial details like that are not handled by this information service. Luckily, Anne is linked to Richard on a credit report, and I got her social security number from that.

Yet before I use it to start hunting her down, I review the properties Richard owns, this time with an eye toward a hiding place for a fugitive. Surely the cops already looked into that, but I guess there's just something about Becks and real estate. I want to check out Kiel's properties for myself.

The house I broke into is a dead-end. Since Richard lived there for the past nine years, I assume that Anne either didn't want it or doesn't need it. Another clue about her perhaps, but nothing new about him.

If it's unrented, the duplex Anne signed over holds promise as a hide-out, but a quick call to an agent in Dad's old real estate office confirms that both halves are occupied. I also ask her about a warehouse Kiel owns on Fourth Street in Landis. She doesn't recognize the address; and when she gets a walk-in customer, I let her go. If I have time, I'll look into that one myself.

The rest of Kiel's holdings are a UPS franchise store located on Main in North Wales, Pennsylvania, a coffee kiosk at the Montgomeryville Mall, and the Audubon Village Inne, an upscale restaurant in a semi-rural area between Valley Forge and Landis. With the possible exception of the Fourth Street address, none of the locations seem at all like a safe spot to lie low.

The clock in the corner of my computer screen reads eleven forty-two, ten minutes later than the last time I looked. Every minute that Kiel remains free cinches my tension tighter. So when the phone rings, my hands jump and so does my heart.

"Hello?"

"Ms. Beck? Lauren Beck?" Now, along with everything else, I'm apprehensive.

"Yes?"

An intake of breath. "Congratulations on your release, Ms. Beck. Would you care to make a comment for the...?"

"Who is this?"

He gives me his name and the television network he represents.

I tell him, "No, thanks," and hang up.

I scarcely finish typing in Anne's social security number before the phone rings again. This time I unplug it from the wall.

Anne's file material is scant compared to her ex-husband's. Just her previous addresses, all in New York, three phone numbers, the apartment complexes she now owns, and one Lexus. Looks like I'm going to have to get out there and beat the bushes.

Karen's hatchback is still in the driveway where I left it the day I was arrested. It starts up grudgingly, so while the engine warms up, I reconsider my first destination. I've got a fondness for the old biddy who spilled her mail all over the yard when I ran out of Kiel's house yelling about a rapist. According to the information service, her name is Mildred Meier, but I decide to let her wait. If Kiel is at the Fourth Street address, and I miss him...Let's just say I don't want to take that chance.

Four forty-nine West Fourth falls in a section of Landis I've never fully explored. Well behind a nursing home (the most reputable establishment in sight), and beside what looks like an abandoned factory, the building Kiel owns sits like a diseased giant–enormous and crumbling. Beneath the steel-meshed windows of the first story, graffiti crawls up the bricks like psychedelic ivy. All the rest of the windows are broken, but I count ten across and four up. A very sizeable amount of floor space, assuming the place still has floors.

All around this lay an empty expanse of uneven asphalt that once served as parking for perhaps a hundred vehicles. Of course, Kiel's year-old Cadillac was found abandoned in the long-term lot of the Philadelphia airport, and nobody knows what, if anything, he's driving now.

I figure if he's inside, he has already spotted me; so I simply park the hatchback a few paces away from the broken glass, tuck my Glock into the front of my waistband, and cautiously leave the confines of the car. A quick scan of the windows, then a rush to the shelter of the building where watching me will prove the most difficult.

In spite of the disrepair, the property has merit. Not very far uphill from the chain-link fence delineating the property line is a busy street, Broad Street of Landis if I gauge correctly. The easy access for potential customers will make the land under my feet ideal for one of those humungous retail facilities like Home Depot or Ikea. Making my way through the trash along the wall, I round the second corner and see what I missed before—a SOLD sign affixed to the front near the building's main entrance. Apparently Abernathy Commercial Properties brokered the deal. Bully for them.

I've been checking doors all along, beginning with a rear loading dock five feet off the ground that once had wooden steps but doesn't anymore. The two ground level doors near where I parked and another on the opposite side are crisscrossed by boards, and the fire escape looks as if it would tumble with a touch.

The only safe entrance is at the front, which possess double doors, once blue but now faded to almost silver. Their brass handles were fitted with a chain and padlock to supplement the usual tumbler and bolt arrangement; hiding here would require camping equipment and the talents of Houdini, first for getting in and then for relocking everybody else out. Never happen.

Concerned about the time I've wasted, I burn rubber on my way out of there.

Twelve minutes later I turn into Mildred Meier's driveway. I have the sensation that I'm being watched; but if Scarp has men staking out the pharmacist's house across the street, I certainly can't see them.

"Mrs. Meier," I greet the Kiel's old neighbor when she finally opens the door a crack. "I'm an investigator with the Amalgamated Insurance Association of North America, and I need to ask you a couple of questions about Anne Kiel." I hand my card through the gap allowed by her chain-bolt. "May I please come in?"

She's a wizened one with a bend in her upper spine. Small wonder she made such a memorable sight hustling uphill to the safety of her house. She examines my card and my face, then asks to see my driver's license. I pass it through and subsequently am shown into a spacious living area carpeted in soft yellow. The furniture speaks of designer help, and recent, too. A curved sectional patterned in black, yellow and bluish green, glass-topped tables and a wall-mounted TV. There are silk daffodils in a Chinese vase on the coffee table and a long wall unit displaying hand-painted plates and crystal. When I compliment Mrs. Meier on the décor, the eyes behind the silver spectacles gleam.

"My granddaughter just graduated design school," she boasts. "This was her senior project."

"You struck a good deal."

"Tell me about it," she agrees. "Sit over there, will you? Where I can see your face." She settles into a swiveling armchair and awaits my first question.

"I don't need much, Mrs. Meier. Just Anne's new name and address, if you have it."

"Can't you get that from the post office?"

"The proper paperwork would take too much time, and I'm afraid I'm in a bit of a hurry," I answer truthfully. "And if Anne didn't leave a forwarding address, it won't pan out anyway."

"Well, I'm sorry to disappoint you, dear, but I don't even know her new name."

"Do you have any idea whether she moved out of state?" That would be bad news for me, because I might not locate her in time to help Scarp find Kiel.

"Oh, no, dear. She married a fellow from Chester county. My daughter saw them having lunch down around West Chester a couple of years ago. Lucy knew what Richard looked like from visiting me, you see; so she realized right away that something funny was going on."

"Two years is a pretty long time. How can you be sure Anne married the West Chester guy and not somebody else?"

Mrs. Meier smoothes her skirt with blue-veined hands. "Because I asked her, dear. That's how."

"You did?"

"Yes, I did. I never liked Richard. He has mean eyes; and when he meets you on the street, he doesn't give you so much as the time of day. So last year when Anne told me she was moving, I asked if that meant Richard was moving, too.

"'No,' Anne says. 'Just me. We're getting a divorce.'

"'That's good,' I told her. 'Because you can do better.'

"'Maybe I already have,' she says, but with a smug little smile as if she thought she was getting away with something.

"Oh?'" I said. "'You mean the pretty boy from down around West Chester?'

"Well, that brought her up short, I can tell you. 'You won't tell Richard, will you?' she says, 'Our lawyers are still working things out.'" Mildred folds her hands and indulges in a self-satisfied smile of her own.

"Way to go," I congratulate her. "Maybe you should be in my business."

My host chuckles. Then she carefully rises from her chair to see me out.

Shaking her hand at the door, I can't resist asking again if there's anything more she can tell me about Anne's whereabouts.

Still holding my hand, she says, "Sorry." Then, "This is important to you, isn't it, dear?"

Suddenly feeling transparent, I confess, "Yes, very."

Looking like a Jedi or perhaps a fairy godmother, Mildred wishes me good luck.

"Thank you," I reply, grateful for the sentiment. "I could use some.

Chapter 34

Nina is out somewhere with Jilly when I get home, and I'm starved. I discover two tuna wraps with spinach and sprouts in the refrigerator, and with minimal regret, I snitch one to eat up at my computer.

My palms are sweating as I access Anne's internet information one more time. Mrs. Meier's belief that Richard's ex-wife is still in Pennsylvania is encouraging, but without Anne's new last name getting her address will be tough. Cross-referencing the entries is my last resort.

The New York addresses won't help. Same with the apartment buildings. Which leaves the three phone numbers I saw before. If they don't pan out, maybe I'll try Klein, the private investigator who screwed up the golf-club case. A P.I. won't have the ethical constrictions of an insurance company, so he can probably squeeze information out of a phone listing without too much trouble. If it comes to that. I'm not eager to spend either the time or the money it will take to hire him.

The first number is most likely the Kiel house phone, because it appears on Richard's list, too.

The second seems to be an old wireless number, also billed to Richard at his current address. Anne probably used it when they were married.

The third number, another cell phone, belongs to one Donald Q. McIntyre.

I take a bite of Nina's sandwich and chew while I enter the new name for yet another search.

When the information fills in, I slap the table and jump from my seat. "I knew it I knew it I knew it," I bubble over.

"Mrs. Meier, you sweetheart, you found me Anne's pretty boy. Woo hoo--Donald Q. McIntyre, 4675 Saddle Lane, Newtown, Chester county."

Now all I have to do is go down there and grill Donald's new wife about her ex-husband. Maybe the slimebag always wanted to go to Colorado, or he loves the pony roundup at Chincoteague but only stays at the So and So Motel. Adores trains—hates to fly. An ex will know all sorts of good stuff like that.

And yes, it's possible—maybe even *probable*—that not one thing Anne knows will be of the slightest use.

I don't care. I'm psyched. Psyched enough to put a message in Scarp's voice mailbox. "Going down to Newtown to talk to Kiel's ex-wife. I'll check in later."

The one person I do not call is the new Mrs. McIntyre. People grow more guarded when they have time to think. And for all I know, Kiel could be hiding out with her. The last place he'd go, right? And the last person who would take him in—granted. But what if that's exactly what the arrogant sonuvabitch expects people to think? Something to keep in mind.

Also, I don't kid myself that Anne will necessarily be home. Mildred Meier was of an age when simply getting from here to there requires some planning. Anne McIntyre, on the other hand, has all sorts of means at her disposal. New hubby's assets include three luxury cars and a pickup with a horse trailer; a condo in Jackson Hole, Wyoming; a house on Shore Drive in Avalon, New Jersey; and a number of other toys I choose to forget. So there's a chance I may need to stake out her house for a while.

With that in mind I change into some comfortable jeans and my best black boots, a nice multicolored cowl-neck sweater and a long black leather jacket with a special inside pocket for the Glock. I also grab Nina's other sandwich.

The directions my laptop produced seem pretty straightforward, and in no time Route 202 South delivers me to one of the wealthiest zip-codes in the nation. I try to concentrate on street signs, but how can I miss the black angus grazing inside a half-mile long white board fence or the row of ancient sycamores with their beautiful dappled bark? Lawns are the size of multiple football fields; houses are mansions. When I finally find Saddle Lane, I drive until I spot a mailbox number, then I drive some more. Finally a discrete sign at the road's edge tells me I've arrived.

One problem. There will be no loitering in front of Donald and Anne's picturesque abode--certainly not in a dusty hatchback with Maryland plates. Might as well just pull into the driveway and take my chances.

A hundred feet straight ahead a very long white barn with an ordinary sloped roof reposes in the winter sun. Beside it an air conditioning unit sits where my Dad would slop his pigs, and there's a riding ring with jumping fences instead of chicken coops. The Hanzel and Gretyl house to my left is all wafers of brown fieldstone that look like gingersnaps glued together with icing. Judging by its placement close to the road, it probably dates back to the time of stagecoaches and four-in-hands.

Two doors--a black one with a shaded patio toward the front and another, possibly for the kitchen, toward the rear. I knock on the former and am soon greeted by a middle-aged blonde woman wiping her hands on an apron.

"My name is Lauren Beck," I tell her. "Is Mrs. McIntyre available?"

The housekeeper or cook, or whoever she is, eyes me up and down, thinks about every possible pro or con, then asks, "Is she expecting you?"

"No, but it's very important that I speak with her. Is she here?"

"She's riding with the Mister."

"Do you mind if I wait?"

"Suit yourself." The door closes.

Okay, the hatchback has a heater, so I'm not going to freeze to death but why not have a little look around first? Check for signs of Richard Kiel perhaps.

I cross the huge parking area and enter the barn. Both ends are open, leaving a center aisle where I can pet the noses of several blanketed horses. Five stalls on either side, all either occupied by animals or totally empty. One tack room, one office like Ronnie's, but larger and locked. I peek through the door's window and see nothing but my own reflection. Nuts. If I were Richard, I would insist on staying in the house anyway. But that would probably be a hostage situation, and the housekeeper wouldn't have been free to answer the door.

At the end of the barn I step out in the open and far, far at the edge of the second field spy two people on horseback. Borrowing a white towel from a hook, I return to open air where the riders can see me wave. Eventually, they pull up and start back.

Soon I see why Mrs. Meier called Anne's new husband a pretty boy--six-foot three, nice even features. Reminds me of Brent W. Cahill, Asshole Extraordinaire.

"Darling, do you know her?" he asks as he helps his wife off her huffing steed, "because I certainly don't."

"No," she admits. "What is it you want?"

I introduce myself, then explain that I'm trying to locate Richard Kiel. "Is there somewhere we might sit down for a few minutes?"

I spoke to Anne, but it's Donald who replies. "My wife hasn't had any contact with him since the divorce became final. I doubt that she can help you. Now if you don't mind..."

"If I were still a cop, I could arrest her as a material witness," I state, "and I can still make that happen. Wouldn't it be easier to simply get this over with? "

Again, to Anne, "Richard is wanted for murder, Mrs. McIntyre. Surely you wouldn't want him to get away with something like that."

The delicate brunette blanches and tries to blink away the shock. "Take the horses to Rodney, Donald," she says in a near whisper. "I'll talk to Ms. Beck in the old den."

"I don't care what bullshit story she makes up about Richard. Don't you see? She has no authority to ask you anything."

"Donald," Anne grasps his arm lightly. "It's all right. I'll be fine."

The man huffs like one of the horses and glares like the devil himself, but he takes the reins and turns the sweating animals toward the barn.

"He's very protective," Anne explains. "He knows how...how Richard hurt me."

"Kiel was abusive?" I blurt. "Physically abusive?"

Anne waves her head no. "Donald just doesn't like me to think about the past. I get...I get upset. That's why I didn't leave a forwarding address. I wanted to, to forget about it all."

"I'm afraid you'll have to make an exception just this once. It appears that he killed..."

"You're serious?" Donald's back, mouth agape. "Richard has been accused of murder?"

"Dead serious, Mr. McIntyre. Plus there are other charges pending against him as well."

"Oh, Lord. I'm sorry. I thought you wanted him for...for personal reasons. An old girlfriend or something."

"No. Nothing like that."

"But why are you here instead of the police?"

"They have their hands full without hunting for a woman without a last name. I had the right kind of experience for the job, so I volunteered."

"But why?"

"That *is* personal. Can we please go inside now? We're wasting too much time."

Donald says something into this wife's ear, shoots me a warning glance, then pivots toward the barn.

Anne gestures me into the rear door, then leads me to a sizeable den full of old furniture. Throwing off her jacket, she flops gracefully onto a sofa that smells of sweaty horse and leather.

"Please sit anywhere you like," she offers, so I pick a no-nonsense straight-backed chair.

"Richard's Cadillac was found in the long-term lot at the Philadelphia International Airport," I open. "Any idea where he might have gone?"

His ex-wife actually smiles. "Who is he supposed to have murdered?" she asks. "Someone you knew?"

"A nurse. And yes, I knew her. Please, every minute we waste..."

"But you're not official. You said so yourself."

"I don't think you appreciate the urgency..."

Anne is taking off her boots, tucking her stockinged feet under her. "Were you seeing Richard? Is that why this is personal?"

So that's what's at play, the power of suggestion. "No," I answer emphatically. "He diluted the chemotherapy drugs given to a friend of mine, and she died as a result. Now will you please tell me where you think he might be?"

Anne McIntyre gawps for a moment. Then she says, "Richard avoids flying."

I sit up straighter. "He's afraid of flying?"

Anne shrugs and reaches for a wooden box containing cigarettes. "His father once worked as a flight attendant. It embarrassed Richard, so he always said his father had been in the airline industry. Later when his dad ran a hamburger joint in South Philadelphia, Richard said he was a restaurateur."

I'm not sure how this is helping me. "So you're telling me Richard doesn't fly?"

"No, I'm just saying he avoids it."

"He would fly if he needed to get out of the country in a hurry?"

"Sure. But not if he could avoid it."

"Okay. Let's go back to the girlfriend idea. To your knowledge, did Richard ever cheat on you?"

"To my knowledge..." she smiles again while she pauses to use the cigarette lighter. "Once or twice. Richard isn't very good with women, but yes, he cheated on me."

"Was he aware that you knew?"

An impish smile from behind some smoke. "He is now."

"Any idea who he saw most recently?"

She waves her head as she leans forward to tap off some ash. "Nobody according to the detective I hired. Richard was a good little boy for at least six months before the divorce...unfortunately." Which explains how he kept the goodies.

"Before, when he was seeing someone, where did they go? Do you have any idea?"

"No, sorry. I never could find out."

"No detective?"

She shrugs again and blows smoke at the sofa. "I was already seeing Donald.

"Tell me," she interrupts herself. "How likely is it that Richard is guilty?" A hint of interest at last, the price evident in the deepened grooves across her forehead.

I choose my words carefully. "Knowing what I know, I would be astonished if he wasn't."

Anne and I regard each other for a moment. Then she resumes breathing and looks away.

"Favorite vacation spots?" I prompt.

"We usually took cruises."

"Any place he particularly wanted to go?"

"Not that I know of."

This isn't getting there fast enough. "Tell me how Richard Kiel thinks, Mrs. McIntyre. Would he appear to leave town and then stay? Would he appear to leave by one means and then use another? You know him better than anyone else—what would he do?"

Anne McIntyre stops smoking and stares over my shoulder. When she meets my eyes again, she says, "Richard is motivated by money. If there was money in it for him, he would stay. If not, I guess he would leave."

"Even if he's guilty of murder?"

Her eyebrows rise and fall. "Don't most people who commit murder think they're going to get away with it?"

"Yes. Yes, they do." Especially if they've framed somebody else. "May I please borrow your phone?"

"Certainly." She hands me a cordless one from the end table beside her.

I use it twice. Three times if you count 4-1-1 for information.

The person I wanted and finally got confirmed Anne McIntyre's assessment of her ex-husband--and mine. Richard would most definitely profit by sticking around until Monday.

Then he would almost certainly disappear.

"You've been a big help," I assure Anne as I stand to go, "and I'm very grateful."

"Just a minute." She catches up with me at the door. "Please, I need to know. Can everybody else find me now? Is this just the beginning?"

"I doubt it." I reach for the door handle.

"But, I mean, how can I be sure? You're here."

Considering the shock I delivered, I owe her a little peace of mind. I turn around.

"A commercial information service linked you to Donald's cell phone number, but unless you skipped out on a debt or left a pile of parking tickets, I doubt that anybody else will bother looking for you that way."

"But Donald's cell phone is for business. I never use it."

"You must have at least once."

Anne frowns while she searches her memory. "Well, maybe once, back before we were married. The electricity was out, and we couldn't use the portable phones. I ordered a pizza."

"And gave the delivery guy Donald's cell phone number, your old name, and this address?"

"I guess I must have."

"That's it then."

"But, but...pizza?"

"Yep. They sell their information to databases." Welcome to the new millennium.

Helpful as Anne McIntyre was, I'm extremely glad to be out of there. A lot of things are coming together in my head, and the highway hum and the softness of the falling twilight conspire to help them gel.

The phone number I got from information had been for the office of Abernathy Commercial Properties, the company that sold Kiel's run-down warehouse in Landis. I didn't expect anybody to be working this late on a Saturday afternoon; but their recording gave me an emergency number, and that put me through to the realtor himself.

Never mind what I said—it was a complete fabrication about an administrative assistant who was supposed to deliver some papers to a settlement, "for a building on Fourth Street," and "is the appointment for Monday or Tuesday?" because I'm eloping this weekend and blah blah blah don't want to come back until I absolutely have to.

Abernathy grumbled until he realized that answering, "Monday at ten," got rid of me quicker.

"Where was that again?" I inquired in character, and he parted with the address of a title company.

Anne McIntyre's eyes were bulging when I hung up, so I shrugged and showed her a grin. "Your ex-husband won't be there," I explained, "but his attorney will. So if we don't catch up with Richard before then, we might be able to use the attorney to find him." But only if, as Anne's insights suggested, Kiel stayed in the area hoping to collect a fat cashier's check before the public finds out he's a fugitive.

I gauge the chances of that at fifty-fifty. Here is a guy who believes that paying taxes on fraudulent profit keeps him above scrutiny. Maybe the same overconfidence left him unprepared for sudden and permanent flight. In that case, a hefty check cashable anywhere would be almost irresistible.

At least that's my theory. The police have everything else covered, so I see no reason not to pursue it. If it doesn't pay off, no harm done.

Yet the more I think about it the more optimistic I become. Each day Kiel remains free will widen the search and render a local hideaway less and less likely, an advantage that might be almost as appealing to Kiel as the money.

And, if I'm right, I might even know where he is.

Chapter 35

So these are the ideas that come together as I drive.

Richard Kiel needs a place to hide where nobody will think twice about his behavior. A place that doesn't require a credit card and maybe not even cash. Food and warmth are a given. This is not a camp-out-in-a-disaster-area kind of guy. I figure he's where he took his girlfriends when he cheated on Anne. I figure he went to the Audubon Village Inne. It's a shame I didn't come to this conclusion sooner, but prior to Anne McIntyre's input like everybody else I was working on the assumption that Kiel was already out of the state, possibly even out of the country.

After Anne helped me focus on the local idea, I also remembered that for an establishment to be called an inn, or "Inne," at least one bedroom must be available to the public. Otherwise, Kiel's place would be called the Audubon Village Eatery, or Restaurant, or Diner. Probably has something to do with faulty advertising. Just because everybody goes there for the filet mignon in puff pastry doesn't mean the bedrooms don't exist.

And what employee would dare question the owner if he chose to use one for his own purposes? None. I once worked for a jerk with the morals of a rabbit on Viagra, but I closed my ears when he made his motel reservations because I needed my job.

These are my thoughts as I speed north on Route 202 toward the territory above Valley Forge Park. A short winter twilight has already ended, and the hatchback's headlights cut through a falling dew that moistens the road. After a brief stint on Route 422, I exit onto a rambling two-lane back road then pull over the first chance I get. I need to bring Scarp up to speed again, and I know better than to do that while I'm driving.

Unfortunately, he isn't answering his cell phone and can't be found at his county office or any of the Landis police stations. I leave messages everywhere, one even with a live person, asking the detective to meet me at the Audubon Village Inne *immediately*, that I'll be waiting. Always best to arrange for backup and be wrong than to go it alone and get hung out to dry.

Tucked into the heavily wooded Pennsylvania countryside among a discreet collection of houses, the Audubon Village Inne is an oasis of light. Painted white with a prominent wrought iron "1709" affixed to the street side, one can easily imagine coaches dropping off ladies at the curb or horses being sheltered in the open shed at the far edge of the parking lot.

About thirty cars are lined up under a twinkling row of trees. I find a slot facing the road and leave the hatchback's motor running while I wait for Scarp or whoever he sends. He has Karen's cell number, which I keep handy in case he wants to alert me to his plans.

After forty-five minutes, I begin to worry that he didn't get any of the messages. Unlikely, but possible. I convince myself to wait a little longer.

Another half an hour and I decide the miserable S.O.B. doesn't trust me or believe me or care about me. He should be here, and he isn't. So what if he's stuck somewhere inconvenient? He should call. He should send a squad car. He should do *something!*

Unless he happens to be busy apprehending Richard Kiel.

Feeling deflated, I make my way into the Audubon Village Inne alone.

The entrance takes a hard left turn into a hall that runs across the front of the building. Low-hung tall windows allow plants to thrive but chill both me and the hostess clutching her cardigan closed at the podium.

"Do you have a reservation?" The woman inquires, showing me a stiff mannequin smile to go with her stiff mannequin hair.

"I'm meeting someone, but I'm early. Mind if I just look around while I wait?" I pretend to admire the main dining room, with its exposed beams and gas fire dancing in the hearth. Twinkle lights and poinsettias all around. Thanksgiving in a week; Christmas in five.

"Perhaps you would prefer to wait in the bar?"

"No thanks. I'll just wander." This displeases the hostess, but what's she going to do?

Beyond her is an intriguing L-shaped hall that might or might not lead upstairs. I don't want to attract the hostess's attention again, so I turn around and peek into the smaller dining room behind me. No fireplace, and only twelve tables—all occupied but one.

I stroll closer to the entrance of the larger room, which has an enormous chandelier and twice as many tables, five of them still ready and waiting. But, of course, the evening is young. I suspect another private dining room either in the back or perhaps on the second floor, because muted cocktail conversation comes from somewhere I can't see.

To my immediate left, just off the hostess's hip is a modest-sized bar. The entrance wall is totally open, and the bartender's work area backs up to the dining room; but the other two closed walls are mahogany paneling topped by mullioned windows overlooking that interesting hall. A narrow door in the back accesses it as well, probably a shortcut to the rest rooms. I go through that way, past the manager's office to the far end of the passage, and here is my staircase. Three feet wide with worn carpet and minimal lighting, your eye slides right past it to the security exit a few feet beyond.

I tiptoe up the stairs into a dark, thirty-foot long hall lined with five doors—the bedchambers from the original old-time inn. Electric candles light each doorway, and a table with the requisite poinsettias brighten the window at the far end.

When I see light seeping out from under Door Number Three, I want to punch the air and cheer. I'm not crazy. Somebody actually is staying here.

A lanky waitress is assembling a tray of drinks at the end of the bar.

"Excuse me," I say as I approach. "I've got a date upstairs with, um, your, um, boss, and I was wondering—did he have dinner yet?"

The woman's expression opens with alarm, but quickly switches to relief. "No he hasn't, and he should. He really should. He's been a bear this whole time. Maybe now that you're here he'll cheer up a little. Nobody wants to go near him."

I pretend to sigh with my own relief but I'm jumping out of my skin. Richard Kiel is here. This whole horrible mess might end tonight.

"Okay, um, what's your name?"

"Randi."

"Okay, Randi, I'm going to make a little confession here. Richard and I, we had a fight—you know how it is. So he isn't exactly expecting me. So I sort of need to know. Is anybody else up there?"

"Oh, hell no. He's all yours, honey." With that she swirls off toward the dining room with the tray of drinks.

Which gives me an idea. I turn to the bartender. "And what's your name?" He's a touch overweight, but cute nevertheless.

"Brian," he tells me with a smile.

"Brian," I repeat, as if I like the sound. "I'm here to visit Mr. Kiel upstairs, and I'd like to surprise him with his favorite drink. You think you could make one for me and put it on a tray?" I slip a ten onto the bar.

"Beefeaters on the rocks? I can manage that," he pushes the ten back toward my hand.

"Thanks."

"Thank *you*," he replies, seconding the waitress's sentiment.

I take the tray and silently ascend the stairs once again. A few steps from Richard's door I set the tray down, fish Karen's cell phone out of my purse, and put it in my jeans pocket—heaven forbid I should have to cross the room to call 9-1-1 if everything goes south—then I take the Glock out of my leather jacket and check the load. Toss my purse and jacket under the poinsettia table. Pick up the tray with my left hand, center myself, and tap on the door to Number Three.

No response.

I tap again. "It's Randi from downstairs, Mr. Kiel," I call out, imitating her voice. "Brian thought you might be ready for another Beefeaters."

I hold the tray with the drink close to the peephole so it's the only thing Kiel will see.

A hesitation, then the sound of the chain bolt being undone. A hand eases the door open while a familiar voice starts to say something.

I miss the words because of the deafening sound in my ears—the mother of all blood rushes brought on by blind fury. I am scarcely aware of dropping the tray, grabbing

Kiel's wrist, and yanking with all my might. I think his head cracked against the doorjamb, because for a second I see his face upside-down and backward. He looks very surprised.

After that—just bits and pieces. I know Kiel pulled me down with him because my hip is bruised. I know I hit him with a ceramic lamp because I can still see it shattering against his head. Either then or later he fell sideways onto a fragile antique table.

For certain I took a foot or a knee to the stomach. And yes, the toe of my right boot is deeply cut and the rear pocket of my jeans is gone. I have a black eye and a lump on the back of my head, countless bruises, and a wrenched back. I've got a three-inch scratch across my cheek, perhaps from a piece of the lamp, and my right elbow is totally black and blue.

I have dreams—nightmares. In them I'm kicking Richard Kiel repeatedly. He is curled on the floor writhing, begging me to stop, but I am deafened by my own voice. *Corinne Wilder,* I shout. *Amy Dion. This is for...*and then I name someone in my acquaintance who died of cancer— *Patty Shields,* or *GeeGee White,* or *Barbara Bates. Herb Ballard, Thomas Rooney,* or *Angela Rittenhouse.* The list is long, every kick a catharsis.

I wake up consumed by guilt, terrified the dream is true. I'm convinced that if tears hadn't blurred my vision I might have kicked Richard Kiel to death.

When the roar finally subsides and real time returns, I become aware of two men and a woman staring down at me—Brian the bartender, another older man, and Randi, the waitress. For a second I think they're there to finish me off, and my hand instinctively goes for my Glock. It's gone, of course, fallen or thrown out of reach by

CURED   **241**

somebody's guardian angel. Otherwise either Kiel or I would surely be dead.

Then my head clears a little, and I think maybe the people are here to help. I hope so, because I hurt all over.

Yet nobody makes a move in my direction, possibly because I'm sitting up and Richard Kiel is not. Randi and the older man circle my outstretched legs and hurry over to examine him. Their employer appears to be a goner, but Kiel groans as together they roll him onto his back.

Face up, I can see that Kiel is a bloody mess, mostly because of the gash on his scalp. Also, his forearm doesn't look right. His breathing is shallow but not labored like Corinne's was. He just has something wrong with his ribs.

"Jesus," the bartender swears as he shies away from the sight. "What'd he do to you?"

The cops arrive then with flashing lights and sirens, also the ambulance the manager had the foresight to order. Kiel requires more urgent attention than I, but fairly soon I do get checked over and bandaged. I'm also given two humongous pain pills for later on. Once again, it seems that I will live to fight another day.

One of the beat cops is young and eager, a smooth-shaven rookie pumped up by the novelty of the "the Audubon Ambush," as the news reports will soon label tonight. Kiel's image was indeed taped to his squad car's dashboard; so he knows exactly who he has, if not precisely why.

I answer his questions with an icepack on my cheek, and eventually the kid simmers down enough for me ask one of my own.

The answer: "Scarp Poletta? Never heard of him." So it seems that the homicide detective elected to ignore my plea.

He shows up just as Kiel is being carried out.

"Hold on a second," he says then walks over and handcuffs the unconscious pharmacist to the gurney. "Catch up with you at Soames," he tells the medics.

A minute later we're alone. Scarp seems to be completely without words, but I'm well into my adrenaline crash, aching to the roots of my hair, and I know exactly what I want to say.

"Where the hell were you?"

Scarp fists his hands on his hips and waves his head in a manner both astonished and annoyed.

"You're kidding, right?"

"Hell, no. I left messages everyplace."

"That was you?" he exclaims. "All I heard was some pushy bitch wanted to buy me dinner."

Chapter 36

No dinner, just lunch on Monday.

Scarp and I spoke on the phone three times yesterday, and he finally confessed that his head had been so totally into a false Kiel spotting in Atlanta that he'd set himself up to misunderstand my message. To be fair, the Atlanta details were persuasive enough that I can't say I wouldn't have made the same mistake. In the spirit of détente I admitted I might have parted with a few more details myself, and we agreed to meet at my favorite eatery, an old-fashioned diner with the stainless-steel façade of an Air Stream trailer. I love their blueberry waffles and bacon any time of day or night, and coffee refills are free.

"Nice shiner," Scarp remarks when he joins me. "Very...colorful." I hadn't bothered trying to cover it with make-up.

He orders a Coke and a San Diego chicken sandwich, then pushes aside his flatware and gives me a breezy, "So what've you been up to?" He means this morning, since our last update was ten o'clock last night.

I stick a straw in my ice-water and tell him I checked on the Taurus. "Forensics still wants to compare Kiel's fingerprints with the ones they lifted from the car." If a suspect's prints aren't on file, sometimes they'll make the comparison after the arrest to strengthen the case. They'd already located the dealer who sold Kiel a duplicate key, which was how he managed to plant my car near the scene of Amy Dion's murder. It makes my head ache to think how well I was framed—even before I was seen in the hallway holding a gun.

After the waitress delivers our food, Scarp remarks, "Speaking of forensics, trace fibers have linked Kiel to Amy's apartment. The case is pretty well made."

"Never in doubt," I joke, and Scarp rolls his eyes.

"So what about you?" I ask as I pick up my fork. "What did you do this morning?" My waffles are perfect, steaming and crisp. Plus they're dripping with syrup and whipped butter.

Scarp sips his Coke then gestures with the tumbler. "I stopped by a real estate settlement and had a chat with an attorney."

"Oh?"

"Oh, yeah. Poor guy didn't have a clue that Kiel was on the run."

"And that was because...?"

"I guess because he doesn't own a police scanner. Also, he's done deals like Fourth Street for Kiel before."

"Like how?"

"Pretty simple, really. He just represented Kiel at the settlement then met him for lunch to hand over the check. Nothing illegal; just a convenience, that's all."

"Bet they weren't meeting anywhere as classy as this."

Scarp lifts the left corner of his mouth, but only slightly. "I believe their reservation was at the Audubon Village Inne."

"I've heard that place has really gone downhill."

"Nah. The owner just went down for the count."

"Seriously. How is Richard?" Not that I care about him. I'm worried about getting slapped with an assault charge.

Scarp waves his San Diego sandwich, causing it to drip on the Formica. "He should have known better than to stand that close to a doorknob," he remarks with only a hint of a smile. "People hit their heads on those things all the time."

"Please don't joke about it, Scarp. Your partner said Kiel has three fractured ribs, a broken arm and a concussion."

"Not to worry. The D.A. and I had a little conversation. He's grateful as all get out for your help..."

"... and understanding?" I'm quick to suggest. "I did spend three whole days in jail."

"That, too. He's still waiting to read your so-called confession, by the way." My chronicle of the past two and a half weeks.

"Why?"

Scarp lowers his eyebrows and smirks out the window. "I think he has trouble falling asleep."

We grin at each other for a moment or two. Scarp appears to be thinking, but I'm not. He's got one of those faces you can just sit there and watch.

"Seen this?" he finally asks, lifting the A section of this morning's *Inquirer* from the bench and pushing it across for me to read. EX-COP EXPOSES MEDICAL FRAUD FROM JAIL.

Sunday's headlines were all about the apprehension of Amy Dion's murderer. Scarp did those interviews himself, giving me credit but not overdoing it; neither of us want to make the D.A.'s job any harder. Anyhow, it's the forensic work done by the police that will insure Kiel's conviction.

However, the chemotherapy fraud is a sensation in its own right, and it seems that all that fuss is going to revolve around me. I've already seen other headlines like this morning's, including ones from national news publications, and they embarrass me no end.

Dr. Shrawder is to blame. Worried about Soames Memorial getting sued, and perhaps even him personally, he refuses to speak to the press—period. I trust—maybe that should be *hope*—he'll be fine since he's the prosecution's star witness regarding the fraud. Yet I sympathize with his caution. "Lawsuit" is a four-letter word to a doctor, especially in Pennsylvania.

"Fess up," Scarp encourages me now. "Did you do anything yesterday *except* talk to the press?"

"As a matter of fact, I got an apartment." Naturally, the sunset one was long gone; but the same real estate agent saw my name in the news. "You're employed by a very solid corporation," she rationalized over the phone, "so I'm confident we can work something out." And, finally, we did.

"Another handyman's special over a garage," I announce without bothering to disguise my pride. No more coattails. No more crutches of any sort. I am completely on my own.

I'm about to ask Poletta how he is with a paintbrush when the voice in my head that monitors such things nixes the idea. I've been spot-checking for vibes, and the man comes off way too friendly and relaxed. In other words, no sexual tension. I'm disappointed, but not surprised. The Audubon Village Inne fiasco was a major clue. He hadn't even asked *who* wanted to take him to dinner.

Our lunch is almost finished, but there's one more item on my agenda. "Scarp," I begin as I set my napkin aside. "I've got a favor to ask."

A panicky "what now?" expression comes and goes, quickly replaced by an open smile. I owe him, certainly, but he owes me, too. I handed him the hugest case to hit Glenndenning county in a long long time.

"Anything," he vows.

"I'd like you to ask the D.A. to indict Kiel for murder."

Scarp's narrowed eyes and wrinkled forehead tell me this wasn't what he expected. "What do you mean?" We both know the pharmacist has already been arraigned.

"Not Amy. I know he'll pay for that. I want justice for some of the cancer patients he killed."

"Corinne?"

"I wish, but I'm afraid her death was too indirect. You've got to pick somebody from Soames's list that should have lived and didn't. I don't care whether you do one person or two hundred and one, but I'd like Kiel's 'depraved indifference' to be seen as the murder, or attempted murder, it really was."

Scarp nods ever so slightly. "Okay," he says. "I'll try. I'm not saying the D.A. will go for it, but I'll do my best."

"Thanks. That's all I ask."

Our conversation gets a little awkward after that. We even remark on the weather. The waitress drops off the check, and Scarp settles up.

We pause outside in the parking lot. I kiss him on the cheek and say, "Tell Rainy hi for me."

Scarp's face actually brightens before he realizes that I've called him out.

"It's okay," I reassure him. "Have a nice life. Get a dog and have babies—the whole nine yards."

He doesn't reply. Instead he looks sheepish and grateful. Probably even more grateful than when I handed over Richard Kiel.

When I arrive back at the office, I'm still congratulating myself on my maturity. I believe I've done a few things right for a change, and I'm allowing myself to feel pretty good about myself, a luxury that doesn't come along all that often.

"Hey, David," I greet my boss when he pops out of his office. "How's it going?"

He hooks a hand around my elbow and turns me around. "Aaron Ashmead wants to see you."

"The big boss?"

"None other."

"Wow!" Since my supervisor's face doesn't give away a thing, I ask what it's about.

"I'm sure he'll tell you," David replies, then escorts me all the way up to the head honcho's corner office without another word.

The view from the top floor is spectacular, a panorama of Pennsylvania countryside ending with a skyline of Landis. Winter is obviously in the wings—snow and mulled wine by the fire and the smell of wet wool. I'm ready. I'm ready for anything.

"Please sit down, Ms. Beck." The Director of Operations for the Eastern Claims Division of the Amalgamated Insurance Association of North America waves me into a leather visitor's chair. He is a Winston Churchill look-alike minus the cigar. Probably read the actuarial tables regarding smoke inhalation. David has already disappeared, silently shutting the door behind him.

"Quite a splash you had in the papers yesterday," Ashmead opens, his delivery telegraphing that he is merely making a comment, as anybody would.

"Yes, sir." Nothing about my black eye?

"In fact you've had two very eventful weeks." If anything, now he seems put out; so perhaps he's aware of my arrest but not my personal loss, which, come to think of it, is probably true.

I try to reply, but the D.O. isn't listening. He's lifted a sheet of paper and is standing there reading it.

After a bit, he looks up and scowls. "The Megan DeMarquess case," he remarks. "It says here you spoke to the victim."

This is what he wanted to see me about?

"Well, yes. I determined that the couple were conspiring to move the case forward to help pay for a baby. I talked them out of the claim."

"You talked *them* out of the claim."

"Yes, sir. Megan DeMarquess rear-ended her boyfriend's car on purpose. I, uh, explained to them that she wasn't covered for that."

"I see. What about this? It says here that you let the air out of Mr. Tanner's tire. Is there anything to that?"

I was positive I hadn't been seen, so how...? Damn. No puncture when Jimmy took it in to get fixed.

"May I ask where you're going with this line of questioning, sir? It seems to me that I've done some good work for the company that you haven't mentioned."

"Such as?"

"I saved AIA one point six million on a fraudulent closed-head injury. A man who was accidentally hit by a falling golf club..."

"Oh, yes. I heard about that." He may have heard about it, but he's not impressed.

"... and what about the fire at the travel agency? I got the ex-wife to admit it was arson."

"Yes, yes. Let me ask you this. How many cases have you cleared in three weeks?"

Not very many. Not enough is what the Director of Operations is about to say.

I jump the gun. "You're firing me? This isn't because I was arrested for murder, is it? Because..." I can go no farther. The injustice of this, this *corporate* decision is threatening to ruin my sunny disposition.

Yet instead of sinking into a pout, I toss a hand and risk a question. "When *Time Magazine* drops by for my interview tomorrow, wouldn't you like me to tell them that I work for AIA?"

Ashmead lifts his Winston Churchill chins a quarter inch. "Tell them whatever you like, Ms. Beck," he says, "*except* that you work for AIA, because that will no longer be true."

Really? After all I...*Really?*

To hell with self-control. I stand up and lean into his personal space. "I solved the biggest medical fraud Pennsylvania has ever seen," I remind him through clenched teeth. "People will be talking about the Kiel trial for months, maybe even years."

Ashmead doesn't flinch, perhaps because he already knows how our meeting will end. His brow develops a puzzled crease, though, as if he's watching me without sound.

So naturally I turn up the volume. "Kansas City..." I heard this from one of the reporters. "... another pharmacist caught diluting chemotherapy drugs. The jury awarded one of the victims—just *one,* mind you—two point two billion dollars,*" and here I really get in the D.O.'s face, "... *two point two **billion** dollars!*"

That brings him to his feet. He inflates his chest and curls his lip into a you-just-don't-get-it sneer.

"And who do you think will be expected to pay that *two point two billion*? Eh? You ever hear of **liability insurance**?"

How can I have forgotten? It is companies like AIA who get tapped for the exorbitant punitive awards. Ashmead can—and probably will—swear on a stack of bibles that he fired me for poor performance, when the truth is that loose cannons like me give him ulcers.

"Do no wrong," David had advised, and finally—finally—I understood.

Tuesday. Chris, the real estate agent with the chipped tooth, is standing just outside her office glaring after me; so I toss her a feeble good-bye as I climb into my sister-in-law's hatchback. We had an uncomfortable couple of minutes back there, but the deposit for the apartment is now safely back in my wallet along with my AIA severance check. Karen's car is loaded low with my stuff, and I've got a country-western station all set to accompany me back down I-95. The weightiest question on my mind right about now is what my sister-in-law will have on hand for lunch.

Future plans? I don't have any yet. Take it easy for a couple months for sure, enjoy my family and the farm. Ronnie says he knows a waterfront pub that's always short on bartenders, so I might do that for a while. You know, sock away some cash while I give this employment problem the consideration it deserves. I'm supposed to have a nice long life ahead of me—on paper at least—so I figure I should take a stab at getting it right.

It's the damnest thing though. When I told the *Time Magazine* reporter I wasn't with any particular company, she said, "Oh, then you're a private investigator." I set her straight, of course. By all accounts, going solo is a tough row to hoe—chancy, boring, lonely. In short, a terrible idea.

I should forget about it, right?

Acknowledgements

Many people contributed to my inspiration and education for this endeavor, and I am most grateful to them all. Dr. Ken Zamkoff, an oncologist and dear friend, started me off with the initial idea. Then kismet put me together with Col. Carol A. Brentlinger of the Commemorative Air Force. We got acquainted over her pumpkin-pecan pie recipe at a football game, and although my baking effort was a disaster, Carol's personal history inspired Lauren Beck's bravery and unique outlook on life, and for that Lauren and I can't thank her enough.

Finding a female insurance investigator was a bit of a trick, but Ginny Greene at the NICB directed me to Special Agent Maureen Gould, whose expertise proved invaluable to me. There is much to be admired in her and those who do her work, and I hope they forgive me for botching it up.

Chief of Police Joseph S. McGuriman of Lansdale, PA, and his Office Supervisor, Cindy Leach, were kind enough to instruct me on the ins and outs of professional law enforcement. They can expect to hear from me again.

I had so much to learn that I tapped many other sources as well. My long-time mentor Harriet Mae Savitz, whose patience with me has always been remarkable, Kathleen DeSouza, Dorinda Shank, Joseph Terry, Cy Young, Rachel Gerrity, Andrea Korn from Sovereign Bank, Bob Wilson, Manager of Larmon Photo, and Victoria Hoeningman, FCLS, Special Investigation Unit, Arson (Allstate Insurance)—each one enriched the book in his or her own special way, and I thank them one and all.

The beautiful cover art, which I adore, was done by Daniel Middleton of Scribe Freelance.

Thanks, too, to my final readers, Mindy Kitei, Earlene Fowler, husband Hench, and especially Robynne Graffam, my superb editor–wise advisors all.

Donna Huston Murray

www.donnahustonmurray.com

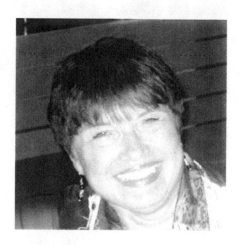

In addition to the seven Ginger Barnes Main Line mysteries
originally published by St. Martin's Press, Donna Huston
Murray has written for MYSTERY SCENE MAGAZINE,
READER'S DIGEST, ECHELON, and REDBOOK. Her
work can also be found in the Edgar-award winning
companion book, THE FINE ART OF MURDER, and the
LETHAL LADIES I and II anthologies by Berkley.
CURED is her first novel of suspense.

Donna and her husband live in the Philadelphia area and
have two adult children.

CPSIA information can be obtained at www.ICGtesting.com
Printed in the USA
LVOW061543140113

315660LV00001B/106/P